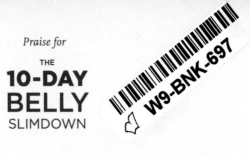

Praise for

THE

10-DAY
BELLY
SLIMDOWN

"The best gift you can give yourself is a slim, beautiful, healthy belly—and in this book Dr. Kellyann, an expert I trust, tells you exactly how to get it."

—MEHMET OZ, MD

"This isn't another gimmicky diet—it's a powerful eating strategy that will take your extra pounds off quickly, safely, and permanently."

—MARK HYMAN, MD,
#1 *New York Times* bestselling author of *Food: What the Heck Should I Eat?*

"*The 10-Day Belly Slimdown* is perfect for those who want to shed stubborn belly fat! What I love is that Dr. Kellyann helps you do it without sacrificing flavor! This is the perfect plan for busy women on the go."

—LAILA ALI,
author of *Food for Life*, TV host, and boxing world champion

"If you're committed to achieving true health, getting rid of dangerous belly fat needs to be your top goal. In this book, Dr. Kellyann shows you how to take those pounds off and keep them off for the rest of your life. And the recipes are awesome!"

—STEVEN MASLEY, MD, FAHA, FACN, CNS, CCD,
author of *The Mediterranean Method*

"Unlike fad diets, Dr. Kellyann's plan is smart and science-based—and in addition to taking off your belly fat, it will make you younger and more beautiful all over."

—NAOMI WHITTEL,
New York Times bestselling author of *Glow15* and *High Fiber Keto*

"Dr. Kellyann is a leader in the weight-loss and anti-aging fields, and she knows her stuff. *The 10-Day Belly Slimdown* is simple, doable, and incredibly powerful. This plan doesn't just take pounds off your belly—it's a serious anti-aging plan that really works."

—ANTHONY YOUN, MD, FACS,
America's Holistic Plastic Surgeon™ and author of *The Age Fix*The

THE
10-DAY
BELLY
SLIMDOWN

**LOSE YOUR BELLY,
HEAL YOUR GUT,
ENJOY A LIGHTER,
YOUNGER YOU**

KELLYANN PETRUCCI, MS, ND

RODALE BOOKS

NEW YORK

The material in this book is for informational purposes only and is not intended as a substitute for the advice and care of your physician. As with all new diet and nutrition regimens, the program described in this book should be followed only after first consulting with your physician to make sure it is appropriate to your individual circumstances. The author and publisher expressly disclaim responsibility for any adverse effects that may result from the use or application of the information contained in this book.

Copyright © 2018, 2021 by Best of Organic, LLC

All rights reserved.
Published in the United States by Rodale Books, an imprint of Random House, a division of Penguin Random House LLC, New York.
rodalebooks.com

RODALE and the Plant colophon are registered trademarks of Penguin Random House LLC.

Originally published in hardcover in the United States by Harmony Books, an imprint of the Random House Publishing Group, a division of Penguin Random House LLC, New York, in 2018.

Library of Congress Cataloging-in-Publication Data
Names: Petrucci, Kellyann, author.
Title: The 10-day belly slimdown / Dr. Kellyann Petrucci, MS, ND.
Other titles: Ten-day belly slimdown
Description: First edition. | New York : Harmony Books, [2018] | Includes index.
Identifiers: LCCN 2017046126| ISBN 9781524762995 (hardback) |
      ISBN 9781524763008 (ebook)
Subjects: LCSH: Reducing diets—Recipes—Popular works. |
    Diet therapy—Popular works. | Weight loss. | BISAC: HEALTH & FITNESS /
    Diets. | HEALTH & FITNESS / Weight Loss. | HEALTH & FITNESS /
    Nutrition.
Classification: LCC RM222.2 .P4963 2018 | DDC 613.2/5—dc23 LC record
    available at https://lccn.loc.gov/2017046126

ISBN 978-0-593-23364-1
Ebook ISBN 978-1-5247-6300-8

Printed in the United States of America

Cover photograph by Keith Major

10 9 8 7 6 5 4 3 2 1

First Paperback Edition

Success is a funny thing. At times, it's easy to believe
it's all about my writing skills, my speaking skills,
or a catchy book cover.

What I've learned is that it's much more than that.
It's about *you*. You giving me the chance to enter your
homes and transform your lives.

I dedicate this book to you, my readers and viewers.
My sincerest thanks, respect, and limitless gratitude to all of
you. It's an honor to play a role in your journey to becoming
slimmer, younger-looking, and healthier *fast* using the
program and principles in this book.

CONTENTS

FOREWORD

Long before I got to know Dr. Kellyann, I was an online fan—and knew that I had to meet this cool, dynamic woman in person.

When we first got together at the Soho House New York in Manhattan, I could see immediately that Dr. Kellyann walks the walk. She radiates positivity and energy. Her skin glows, her eyes sparkle, her hair shines, she looks healthy.

What I love most about Dr. Kellyann is that she truly is all about beauty from the inside out. She understands the connection between being healthy on the inside and looking gorgeous on the outside—and she gives you the tools you need to achieve both goals naturally.

A gifted clinician, Dr. Kellyann has guided thousands of weight-loss transformations during her twenty-four years as a medical practitioner—as well as tens of thousands more through her *New York Times* bestselling book, *Dr. Kellyann's Bone Broth Diet*. Now she's back with an innovative, results-driven plan to slim your belly fast.

I'm a fan of really clean, delicious food, and Dr. Kellyann's plan lets you eat fabulous food while getting rid of belly fat. And as a makeup artist, I'm excited that this diet loads your skin with beautifying collagen as it works to give you a more defined waistline.

To me, beauty is confidence. We are all works in progress. While some people are born confident, for most of us that takes some work. We all want to feel and look good and be comfortable in our own skin. Trust in Dr. Kellyann's method to offer the inspiration and tips that will help you become the best version of yourself from the inside out.

Bobbi Brown
Founder of Bobbi Brown Cosmetics and bestselling author of
Bobbi Brown Beauty from the Inside Out

KISS YOUR BELLY FAT GOODBYE!

You're longing to wear skinny jeans. You're aching to wear slinky dresses. You're tired of hiding your muffin top under a beach cover-up or a baggy shirt. And you're fed up with your big belly making you feel old and unattractive.

Well, you know what? If you want a beautiful belly, *you can have it*. In this book, I'm going to show you how to get lean, sculpted abs that will make strangers envy you and your friends ask, "What's your secret?"

Here's my promise: If you follow my plan, you're going to lose your belly fat. You're going to stop hiding and start strutting. You're going to smile when you see yourself naked in the mirror. You're going to go from invisible to insufferably smug—and I'm going to take you there.

And that's not all. In addition, you're going to *take control over* your belly. If you're tired of being bullied by your gut—tired of constant bloating, gas, and constipation—I'm going to show you how to take command. You'll become a *"belly boss,"* and from this point on, your gut will take orders from you.

Want more? I'm also going to tackle the inflammation that makes your *inner belly* old and sick, so you won't just look younger on the outside—you'll *be* healthier on the inside. In addition, I'm going to load you with nutrients that beautify your skin, hair, and nails and heal your joints while they melt away your belly fat. And I'm going to balance your hormones so your uncontrollable cravings become history.

As a result, your friends won't just envy your gorgeous belly . . . they'll wish they had your energy, your youthfulness, and your ability to walk away from that doughnut box without a second look.

While this may seem like a quick-fix diet, it's not. This is an inflammation-blasting, blood sugar–balancing, gut-healing program that will slim your belly and make you look younger and feel healthier.

I know these are big promises, but trust me: I'm up to the job. I'm a weight-loss specialist with more than twenty years of amazing transformations under my belt, and I've also helped tens of thousands of people lose weight through my books and my appearances as a regular contributor on *The Dr. Oz Show.*

In addition, I currently work with some of the biggest names in Hollywood and New York City—men and women who need to look *perfect* onstage or on-screen. For these celebrities, an extra inch on the waistline can kill a career (and gas and belly bloat are out of the question). Every single day, these stars' bellies need to be flawless.

What's more, these celebs can't take the risk of doing diets that leave their skin dry and wrinkly or wreak havoc on their hair and nails. And they can't afford to get derailed by cravings that could potentially put them out of work. So they need a diet that makes them beautiful all over, controls their appetite, and puts them at the top of their game.

I have to work magic to keep these stars beautiful inside and out—and I do. Moreover, I get results *fast.* While hundreds of thousands of people have lost weight on my 21-Day Bone Broth Diet, the celebrities I work with don't always *have* twenty-one days to slim their bellies. Frequently, they have a big event coming up quickly—a movie shoot, a concert tour, a TV special—and they don't have three weeks to get a beautiful belly.

It's not only celebrities who need to slim their bellies fast, either. Many of my patients are up against a deadline, too—a wedding, a class reunion, a beach vacation. These people tell me, "Help, Dr. Kellyann—I need to lose this weight *now!*"

That's why I've found a way to take off up to ten pounds of belly fat in just ten days. That's right—ten days. Now I'm going to work the same magic on you. Give me ten days, and I'll give you a slimmer belly.

What's my secret? A revolutionary diet based on state-of-the-art research showing that simply shrinking your eating window (meaning the hours during which you eat) can send your weight loss into the stratosphere. Think of this as *mini-mini-mini* fasting.

We're going to combine this strategy with two other powerful fat blasters—meals loaded with collagen and other delicious fat-burning superfoods, and lots of rich bone broth to nuke your cravings—to make you burn belly fat faster than you ever thought possible.

And you know what? I'm not *just* going to get you into smaller clothes. I'm also going to help you look and feel younger, happier, healthier, and more confident. And then I'm going to tell you how to stay that way for the rest of your life.

Why Losing Your Belly Is Life Changing

Getting rid of ugly belly fat won't just change your wardrobe. It's going to change your life.

Why? First of all, there's something about having slim, toned abs that gives you a glow—a new sense of self-respect. It makes you feel stronger, more beautiful, and just plain *fabulous.*

When you slim down your belly, you'll stop concealing your figure and start flaunting it. You'll wear fun clothes that show off your body. You'll walk down the street as if you own it and enter a room with "Look at me" written all over you. And the gorgeous skin, hair, and nails you'll get from this diet will make you even *more* full of yourself.

But that's not all! When you kiss bloat and constipation goodbye, you'll go from sluggish to supercharged. You'll perform better at work, at home, and (dare I say it?) in bed. And when your joints start to heal—another fantastic bonus of this diet—you'll get that spring back in your step.

And that's just the beginning! When you lower your "belly age," you'll speed up your metabolism, reduce your inflammation, and transform every cell in your body. Your heart will work better. Your cholesterol and triglycerides will improve. Your blood sugar will go down. You'll lower your risk of heart disease, stroke, diabetes, and cancer. Your doctor will congratulate you instead of laying a guilt trip on you. (When's the last time *that* happened?)

And finally, when you kick those cravings, you will be in control of your weight forever. Yes, *forever. F-O-R-E-V-E-R.*

So you're not just going to lose your belly fat. You're going to look and feel like a whole new you.

The Icky Facts About Belly Fat

If you want still more reason to get rid of your belly fat, let's talk for a minute about just how sick that fat is making you—because it's not a pretty picture.

If you have excess belly fat, chances are that you are aging far faster than you need to be. You know why? Because even fat cells have to be healthy! When they aren't, they release a cascade of hormones that can make you very sick and age you prematurely.

To understand why belly fat is so dangerous, you need to know how your body stores calories in its fat cells. Researchers used to think that we had a set number of fat cells in our bodies, and as we stored more and more calories, the existing cells simply got bigger (along with our waistlines), and no harm done. In short, it seemed we had an almost limitless ability to store excess calories effectively (if perhaps unattractively). Wrong!

It turns out that belly fat is actually very active, and every year we recycle about 10% of our total belly fat cells.[1] Some of us are lucky; our fat cells behave normally because we can make lots of new cells to store excess calories. But others of us can't make enough, so our existing fat cells get larger and larger. Unfortunately, we now know that this is not without consequences.

When fat cells get larger, everything goes bonkers inside these cells, and they become extremely unhealthy. Picture a fat cell as a house: Everything works great if it's just your family living in that house, right? But imagine what would happen if all your friends and your entire extended family moved in, as well! Stressful? You bet.

This is exactly what happens inside your belly fat cells. The stress of excess storage leads these cells to release pro-inflammatory hormones that wreak havoc throughout your entire body. This increases your risk for autoimmune diseases such as lupus and Hashimoto's thyroid disease. It also increases your risk of developing cancer and dementia and of having a stroke or heart attack.

Moreover, unhealthy fat cells start to resist insulin, and insulin is one of the most important hormones in your body. One of its biggest jobs is to hold hands with sugar molecules and help usher sugar into your cells so they can use it as energy. Insulin also interacts with your belly fat, telling fat cells to release energy in a controlled fashion.

But unhealthy fat cells resist rather than respond to insulin. They treat insulin like an unwelcome guest knocking at the door. This leaves your fat cells with only one choice: to store more calories and get even unhealthier.

Eventually, your belly fat cells reach a tipping point and start to "leak," releasing large amounts of molecules called *free fatty acids* into your bloodstream. These free fatty acids get deposited in your heart, liver, and pancreas, causing those organs to age prematurely. This, in turn, leads to cholesterol problems, diabetes, and vascular dysfunction.

And that's not all. Did you know that the health of your belly fat also helps determine whether or not your immune system works well overall? Research shows that excess belly fat can actually blunt your immune system, causing you to get sick more often.

When you take off that extra belly fat on my 10-Day Belly Slim-down, you're going to take enormous pressure off your fat cells. These cells will then start to release anti-inflammatory hormones (happy hormones) that promote healing and protect your heart and brain. So you won't just look good; you'll no longer be aging at an accelerated rate.

In short, this is actually far more than a lose-your-belly-fat plan; it's really an *anti-aging* plan. And it's far more powerful than Botox, face-lifts, and night creams, because it makes you younger from the inside out.

NOTE: You can measure the health of your fat cells using advanced biomarker testing. Adiponectin and leptin are two hormones whose levels you can check yourself through direct lab testing. In most states, you can order these tests online, visit a local blood draw station, and receive your results via secured e-mail within one week. One resource I recommend is: YourLabWork.com/Dr-Kellyann.

My Philosophy

If you know me already, you know that I don't just want you to get slim and gorgeous. I want you to be happy and healthy, too.

That's why this diet is a safe, nutrition-packed program—not a risky, quick-fix plan. And it's why my plan will motivate you to slim your belly now *and* keep the weight off forever.

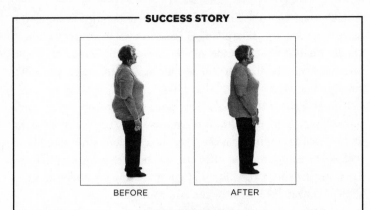

BEFORE AFTER

BEA WILSON

WEIGHT LOST: 13.4 POUNDS | BELLY INCHES LOST: 5.5

Who says you can't lose weight after menopause? At sixty-eight years old, Bea had the most impressive results of anyone in our test group! She found it more challenging than did many of the younger participants, but she stuck it out. Now she says, "I've lost weight, decreased pain and inflammation, my skin is clearer, and I feel really good!"

Forget About "I Can't"

If you're like most people, you've heard four myths about belly fat. In fact, you may have heard them from your own doctor. These myths lead straight to inaction—so before we get started, I want you to get them out of your head right now. Here they are:

- "Belly fat is part of aging—accept it."

- "If you've had a baby, you'll never have great abs again."

- "Belly fat is hormonal. You can't fight it."

- "You can't diet or exercise belly fat away."

All of this is, to put it politely, *crap*.

Let's start with the first myth: that you're doomed to develop a fat belly as you age. Take a look at me. I'm over 50, and my waist is smaller than it was a decade ago. I've helped thousands of people lose their belly fat in their thirties, forties, fifties, and beyond. It's simply a matter of knowing what to do.

Oh, and about that pregnancy myth? If you're struggling with post-delivery belly fat, I know it feels as if you've been cursed for eternity by the pregnancy witch. But when you follow my plan, those inches are going to come off, and your belly is going to get firm. Trust me: I've had two kids, and I got my slim belly back—and I've shown thousands of other moms how to do it, too.

Now, let's talk about those hormones. *Yes*, the hormonal changes you go through as you age can put weight on your belly. That's true (and I'll talk about this later). But my diet is going to change your hormones in ways that make you burn fat faster.

So forget about those myths, because you *can* lose that belly fat. What's more, you don't need to take my word for it! To evaluate the effectiveness of my diet, I enrolled a test group run by an independent clinician. (You'll see many stories from test group participants throughout book.) Here are the participants' results after just ten days:

- They lost up to 13.4 *pounds*.

- They lost up to 5.5 *inches* around their bellies.

Moreover, the benefits of the diet went far beyond weight loss. Here's what else participants reported:

- Their food cravings disappeared.

- They had better skin, less joint pain, more energy, better sleep, less belly bloating and discomfort, less acid reflux, and more beautiful hair (including fewer gray hairs!).

- Their blood sugar improved, and one participant was able to discontinue taking insulin altogether.

So kiss the "you can't" myths goodbye. You *can* get a beautiful belly—and if you follow my plan, you *will*. In addition, you'll get the other awesome bonuses I've promised: less bloating and gas, healthier skin, thicker hair, happier joints, and lifelong control over your cravings.

How are you going to work all this magic? That's what we'll talk about next.

PART I

THE BASICS OF THE 10-DAY BELLY SLIMDOWN

Are you ready to go from hiding your belly to showing it off? Here's how my 10-Day Belly Slimdown is going to transform your belly from fat and bloated to flat and beautiful.

HOW I'M GOING TO BLAST YOUR BELLY FAT ... *FAST*

A re you sick and tired of your belly fat? Frustrated with diets that don't take it off? Angry that you don't look the way you want to look and can't wear the clothes you want to wear?

Then you're in the right place, because *I'm going to free you from that fat,* and I'm going to do it *fast.*

I've spent over twenty years showing people how to do the impossible: take off stubborn belly fat. That's a long time, and *I know what works.* What's more, as a specialist, I put my entire focus on weight loss and delaying aging. So unlike your regular doctor—who may well assume that 90% of patients will fail at losing weight, and is totally resigned to that—I need to maintain a success rate of virtually 100%. Otherwise, I'm out of a job.

Moreover, as I said earlier, I work with world-famous celebrities who can't take a gamble on a diet that might not work. These celebs have millions of dollars on the line, and they need to *know* that they'll be camera-ready. This means that for me, failure simply isn't an option.

So I don't kid around—and I don't waste time with anything that's ineffective. That's why this diet is different—and why it's going to work.

How I take the pounds off the stars . . . and how I'll take them off your belly, too

Right now, I'm going to introduce you to the three powerful core strategies of my 10-Day Belly Slimdown. Separately, each of these strategies will melt pounds off you. Put them all together, and you're going to *nuke* your belly fat so fast your head will spin.

I've used this diet to take pounds and inches off everyone from Grammy Award–winning singers and New York celebs to regular folks who want to turn heads at a wedding or class reunion. It works, it works *fast*, and it leaves you healthier and younger-looking from head to toe.

What's more, this is an *appetite-control* diet. It's designed to minimize your cravings, so you'll maximize your results.

After guiding thousands of transformations over my career, I've targeted the three most powerful ways to take fat off your belly incredibly fast. Here they are:

- A compressed eating window (think *mini-mini-mini* fasting)—the number-one biggest secret to rapid belly-blasting

- Bone broth "burning" and bone broth "loading"—to quench your cravings and melt off pounds

- Beautifying, fat-melting, gut-healing collagen and other "SLIMgestion" foods, herbs, and spices—superfoods that will optimize your digestion and kick your metabolism into overdrive

Separately, each of these strategies is dynamite. On the 10-Day Belly Slimdown, we're going to *combine* them into a triple punch to achieve incredible results in just ten days. Here's a closer look at how we're going to melt that fat off your body.

STRATEGY #1: WE'RE GOING TO SHRINK YOUR EATING WINDOW

Right now, I'm guessing that you don't give much thought to the timing of your breakfast, lunch, and dinner. After all, what matters isn't *when* you eat but *what* you eat, right?

Well, surprise: As it turns out, the timing of your meals may actually matter *more* than the foods you choose. In fact, as you're about to discover, simply shortening your eating window is *the most powerful weapon you have against belly fat.*

We've known for years, of course, that fasting is a magical way to burn fat off fast. In fact, people who fast intermittently lose weight much more quickly than people who diet but don't fast.

Now, however, we're discovering something even more remarkable. It turns out that you don't need to fast for long periods to get results. Simply moving your daily meals a few hours closer together will help keep those extra pounds off—and that's true *no matter what you eat.* This idea sounds crazy, but there's hard science behind it.

In 2012,[1] scientists at the Salk Institute for Biological Studies in California compared mice that had access to food all day long to mice that ate only during an eight-hour window. Both groups of mice ate a high-fat diet, with about 60% of their calories coming from fat.

(One note here: Soon I'm going to tell you why you need to include several servings of healthy fats in your diet each day to stay slim. This method is not comparable at *all* to the high-fat diet used in this study. Studies like this one load up animals with tons and tons of unhealthy fats. That would be like me telling you to eat a two-pound tub of margarine at each meal, rather than a few teaspoons of olive oil.)

So . . . what happened in this experiment? Over one hundred days, the mice that ate all day got fat and developed high cholesterol, high blood sugar, and liver damage. But how about the little guys that ate for only eight hours each day? They weighed 28% less than the other mice and were still healthy.

Megumi Hatori, a coauthor of the study, said, "For the last fifty years, we have been told to reduce our calories from fat and to eat smaller meals and snacks throughout the day. We found, however, that fasting time is important. By eating in a time-restricted fashion, you can still resist the damaging effects of a high-fat diet, and we did not find any adverse effects of time-restricted eating when eating healthy food."

In a follow-up study,[2] the same researchers fed mice one of four diets: high-fat, high-fructose, high-fat plus high-sucrose, and regular mouse chow. Some mice in each group got to eat all day; others had to eat during a nine-, twelve-, or fifteen-hour window. All of them ate *the same number of calories*, no matter what their eating window was.

This time, the study lasted thirty-eight weeks. At the end, the mice that ate the bad diets within a nine- or twelve-hour window still had their slinky little bodies (even though the researchers let some of them "cheat" on the weekends). The other mice, however, were pudgy little sickos. Moreover, the mice that got fat on the unrestricted schedule lost weight when the researchers began restricting their eating window.

Satchidananda Panda, who led both studies, said, "Time-restricted eating didn't just prevent but also reversed obesity. That was exciting to see."

Shortening your eating window won't just help you stay slim; it'll also help you *get* slim. In a more recent study, Panda and his team asked eight overweight participants who normally ate for more than fourteen hours each day to reduce their eating windows. The researchers report that when these people shrank their eating windows to ten to eleven hours daily for sixteen weeks, "they reduced body weight, reported being energetic, and [experienced] improved sleep."[3]

Want more evidence of the powerful effects of reducing your eating window? Here's what other researchers are reporting:

- A 2017 study involving overweight men and women found that time-restricted eating—in this case, eating only between 8:00 a.m. and 2:00 p.m.—increased fat burning and reduced hunger swings. It also improved *metabolic flexibility* (more on this on page 177), which is the body's ability to switch between burning sugar and burning fats.[4]

- In an eight-week study testing the effects of a short eating window on athletes, researchers assigned thirty-four men who did resistance training to a restricted-eating-window group or a nonrestricted group. They found that even though time-restricted eaters ate the same number of calories as participants with longer eating windows, they decreased their fat mass while their lean muscle mass stayed the same. In addition, their blood glucose, insulin concentrations, and markers for inflammation dropped.[5]

- In a study using a mouse model of postmenopausal obesity, researchers found that despite eating the same high-fat diet as mice with unlimited access to food, mice on a restricted-eating schedule experienced rapid weight loss and exhibited less insulin resistance over time. Time-restricted eating also reduced the severity of fatty liver (a dangerous problem that's currently epidemic in the United States).[6]

- Another study tested the effects of time-restricted eating on "middle-aged" mice. They found that time-restricted eating without any calorie restriction helped alleviate the negative effects of an unhealthy diet on body weight and glucose tolerance.[7]

What's more, the benefits of giving your body a break from food go well beyond weight loss. Science shows that fasting helps keep your brain healthy, improves your insulin sensitivity, lowers your stress, helps you sleep better, improves your hormone production, enhances the function of your mitochondria (the energy factories in your cells), and even helps you live longer. In addition, new research shows that a "fast-mimicking" diet can lower blood glucose dramatically (helping to prevent diabetes) and reduce production of IGF-1, a hormone linked to aging and disease. Mice eating the fast-mimicking diet developed fewer tumors as well.[8] Recent research also indicates that restricting your eating window to fewer hours in the day can lower your risk for breast cancer.[9]

All this makes perfect sense when you think about it. Our genes are nearly identical to the genes of our early ancestors, and they ate only during daylight hours—not at night. (It's hard to find that leftover mastodon leg in the dark when you don't have candles or lightbulbs!) Our bodies are biologically wired for long food-free stretches, and they *need* this time to metabolize our food and clean out toxins. When we cheat them out of this fasting phase, we get fat and sick.

The take-home lesson here is simple: *When* you eat truly is as important as *what* you eat. This is a revolutionary finding that is transforming the way experts think about weight loss, health, and food. And it's why in this diet, you're going to shorten your eating

YES . . . YOU *CAN* SURVIVE SKIPPING BREAKFAST!

I bet you've heard all your life that eating breakfast is all-important. If you skip this meal, many people say, you'll wind up gorging for the rest of the day and packing on pounds.

Well, guess what: That's not true.

A few years ago, a group of researchers decided to take a closer look at this claim. Searching the literature, they scrounged up every relevant study they could find.

And guess what—they discovered that there's *no* good evidence to support the idea that skipping breakfast makes you fat. In fact, they went so far as to call the science behind the claim "distorted."[10]

The *New York Times* summarized the researchers' findings, saying that "only a handful of rigorous, carefully controlled trials have tested the claim . . . and generally they conclude that missing breakfast has either little or no effect on weight gain, or that people who eat breakfast end up consuming *more* [italics mine] daily calories than those who skip it."[11]

So put this myth in the "busted" file. In reality, reducing your eating window by skipping breakfast is one of the best weight-loss tricks in the world.

window dramatically. Basically, you're going to eat two daily meals—lunch and dinner—within a seven-hour window.

Now, before you panic, let me tell you this: *You won't be hungry.*

Let me repeat this: YOU WON'T BE HUNGRY.

That's because during both your fasting window and your eating window, you're going to be loading up on luscious bone broth. And that's what we'll talk about next.

STRATEGY #2: WE'RE GOING TO ADD THE POWER OF BONE BROTH "BURNING" AND BONE BROTH "LOADING"

Bone broth is the secret I've used to slim down tens of thousands of people on my Bone Broth Diet—and now it's going to do the same thing for you. That's why I call it my "liquid gold."

In the morning and between your two meals, you're going to drink cups and cups of this gorgeous broth. Here's a basic overview (I'll give you the details in the next chapter):

- In the morning, you'll drink bone broth enriched with fat-burning herbs and spices. This is the broth "burning" phase, and it will melt the fat off you like magic. This is where most of your belly-blasting will happen.

- In the afternoon, between your meals, you'll drink bone broth loaded with detoxifying, fiber-rich vegetables. This is the broth "loading" phase, and it will cleanse your body and load you up with satisfying fiber to keep you regular, eliminate cravings, and banish the bloat.

Now, let's talk about this bone broth—because it's *awesome.*

I'm betting that you know a little about bone broth already. Maybe you heard Laura Prepon calling it "the fountain of youth" or saw Salma Hayek extolling it as "the Botox alternative." Maybe you heard Gwyneth Paltrow and Kourtney Kardashian singing its praises or caught Shailene Woodley saying that it's "everything." If you live in a big city, you've probably even passed pricey cafés selling it for nine or ten dollars a mug.

Well, guess what. I was doing bone broth *before* bone broth was cool. In fact, I've been prescribing it to my patients for decades, because it's the biggest key to rapid weight loss.

If you haven't tried bone broth, it's nothing like that thin, boring broth in a can. Bone broth simmers for hours and hours, releasing deep nutrition that satisfies your hunger on the cellular level. As a result, you can go for hours between meals without ever feeling deprived. That's why you'll be able to effortlessly reduce your eating window on this diet.

But bone broth does much, much more than simply quench your cravings. Here are three more reasons it's weight-loss magic:

- It's loaded with *gelatin* that soothes and heals your gut. Later, I'll tell you how an inflamed, leaky gut ages and sickens your belly, packing pounds onto it. When you soothe that leaky gut with gelatin—I compare it to rubbing aloe vera on a sunburn— you help it heal, making it healthy and strong again.

- It's rich in the amino acid *glycine*, a powerful inflammation fighter that also flushes fat-promoting toxins from your body.

- It's mostly water, so it keeps you hydrated, boosting your body's ability to burn fat. A study published in the *Journal of Clinical Endocrinology and Metabolism* found that drinking 500 milliliters of water—equivalent to about 17 ounces—increases the metabolic rate by 30% in healthy men and women.[12]

So when you drink bone broth, you satisfy your cravings, heal your gut, fight inflammation, burn fat faster, take years off your inner belly, and cleanse toxins from your body. How's that for belly-fat-blasting magic? It's easy to see why bone broth is a centerpiece of both my 21-Day Bone Broth Diet and my turbocharged 10-Day Belly Slimdown.

And guess what: This fabulous food doesn't just make you lose weight like crazy. You'll also get these bonuses:

- Bone broth is loaded with the building blocks of skin-smoothing *collagen*—so while you're shrinking your belly, you'll be erasing lines and wrinkles, as well. (You'll also get a big dose of wrinkle-blasting collagen elsewhere in this diet—more on that shortly.)

- The *glucosamine* and *chondroitin* in bone broth are the same nutrients many doctors use to treat arthritis. One of the most frequent comments I hear from people drinking bone broth is, "My joints feel so much better!"

- The *magnesium* and *glycine* in bone broth are calming and relaxing, so you'll sleep better and feel less stressed during the day.

All this is why I tell my patients to drink bone broth every day *forever*. You can't do anything—*anything*—better for your health *and* your waistline. And right now, it's going to strip that fat off you fast.

So now you know two of my potent belly-blasting strategies. Now let's look at number three.

STRATEGY #3: WE'RE GOING TO LOAD YOU UP WITH SLIMMING, BEAUTIFYING COLLAGEN AND OTHER "SLIM-GESTION" FOODS

For the next ten days, you're going to eat the most powerful belly-fat-burning foods on the planet. These foods are going to slim, cleanse, and heal your gut. At the end of ten days, you're going to feel like a whole new you, with a flat, beautiful belly.

Let me introduce you to my SLIM-gestion superfoods:

FAT-MELTING, AGE-DEFYING COLLAGEN

People are going absolutely gaga for collagen these days. Watch the news, and you'll hear Jennifer Aniston and other celebrities swearing by it, and you'll see people flocking to buy Jamba Juice's collagen smoothies.

Why is collagen all the rage right now? First of all, it's one of Mother Nature's most powerful fat-melting foods. Collagen has the same gorgeous nutrients as the gelatin you get from bone broth, in a highly concentrated and assimilable form. Like bone broth, it heals your gut and fights inflammation, so your extra pounds fall right off.

And that's not all. The amino acids in collagen build strong, lean muscle, sculpting your core. And collagen fills you up and eliminates cravings, which is why you're going to indulge in a rich, creamy, sinfully delicious collagen shake every single day on this diet.

But collagen isn't just a diet friend. It's a diet friend *with benefits*.

Here's the story. After the age of twenty, you start to lose about 1% of your body's natural collagen each year. That's bad news, because without enough collagen to keep your skin strong, you start to develop wrinkles, sagging, and cellulite.

Sadly, most diets make matters even worse, leaving people looking still older and wrinklier. That's because they deprive people of the nutrients (such as collagen) that protect and strengthen skin.

Well, trust me: That's not going to happen on this diet! Instead, you're going to add a powerful collagen fix to your diet every single day, making you *younger-looking* and *less wrinkly*.

Skeptical? Here's just some of the research showing that you truly *can* eat your wrinkles away by taking a collagen supplement:

- One group of researchers found that women taking oral collagen exhibited "a statistically significant reduction of eye wrinkle volume" in just weeks.[13]

- Another study reported that collagen offers strong protection against sun-induced skin damage and photoaging.[14]

- In a third study, participants using collagen had firmer skin and reported less skin dryness, fewer wrinkles, and a reduction in the depth of their nasolabial folds (laugh lines).[15]

I see results like this in my practice all the time. Patients who are initially hesitant to try my diet because they're afraid it will age them are totally over the moon when they see how moist, dewy, and smooth their skin becomes.

And remember—collagen will give you stronger skin *everywhere*. While it's blasting those wrinkles, it'll also fight that cellulite on your butt and thighs by firming and tightening the skin in these areas. So your friends won't just admire the beautiful belly you'll have after ten days. They'll also whisper behind your back: "Did she have work done?"

And guess what: I'm not done yet. Collagen also strengthens your hair, making it thicker and glossier. A two-part research project involving gelatin (basically, the cooked form of collagen) found that "the most dramatic effect of supplementing the normal diet with 14 grams of gelatin daily was an increase in hair diameter averaging 9.3% in the first study and 11.3% in the second study."[16] The researchers also reported, "Approximately 70% of the subjects in both studies showed increases in hair diameter ranging from 5% to 45%." No thickening shampoo in the world is going to give you results like those.

Want more? Collagen helps strengthen your fingernails. According to researchers, gelatin (again, simply the cooked form of collagen) "increases significantly the hardness of fingernails and apparently improves nail defects in normal subjects."[17]

So you can see why I want you to drink that collagen-rich shake every single day (and why I recommend that you keep up the collagen habit even after your diet is over). In addition to making you slimmer, it's going to give you a makeover *all over*!

BEAUTIFUL PROTEINS

During your diet, you're going to eat clean, natural proteins such as salmon, shrimp, steak, chicken, turkey, lamb, and eggs. These proteins are packed with fat-fighting nutrients, including choline, conjugated linoleic acid, and omega-3 fatty acids, and they're rich in the amino acids that build lean muscle.

VIBRANT VEGGIES

Every day, you're going to load up on gorgeous greens. These foods will fill you up and blast your bloat. They'll also supercharge your cells with phytonutrients that cleanse your body, rev up your metabolism, and blast your belly fat. And they'll give you a big dose of fiber, which can moderate your hunger so you are able to say no to temptation.

FAT-BATTLING GRAPEFRUIT AND BERRIES

I've cut nearly all fruit from this diet because it raises your blood sugar, and that can translate into more belly fat. But two fruits have such amazing fat-burning effects that I want you to eat them every day.

The first is grapefruit, which I want you to include in your diet *unless* it interferes with any medications you're taking (more on this later). Here's why:

- Grapefruit contains a compound called *nootkatone*, which stimulates your metabolism and ramps up your fat burning.

- Animal research shows that grapefruit juice has more powerful weight-loss effects than sibutramine[18] (a diet drug that's now banned)—and, unlike sibutramine, it's good for you!

Berries also punch above their weight when it comes to burning fat. Here's a look at the magic they work:

- Blueberries help burn off abdominal fat and keep your blood sugar under control.[19]

- Strawberries reduce your insulin levels after a meal.[20] (That's important because, as you'll recall, excess insulin leads to insulin resistance—and that leads to more belly fat.)

- Raspberries can protect against visceral fat[21]—and they help activate a hormone called *adiponectin*, which can improve your insulin balance.[22]

In addition, grapefruit and berries are rich in fiber, so they help fight cravings. And berries satisfy your sweet tooth, so they'll help you steer clear of cookies, ice cream, and other diet wreckers.

HIGH-POWERED HERBS AND SPICES

On this diet, you'll load your meals with SLIM-gestion herbs and spices. These foods may be small, but trust me, they're mighty.

Some of these herbs and spices are *thermogenic*, meaning that they turn up your body heat and rev up your metabolism. Others are *adaptogens*—substances that help your body adapt to stress. Still others fight bloat, lower inflammation, cleanse your system, and fight aging.

SLIMMING FATS

Each day on your diet, you'll eat two servings of luscious, healthy fats. *Yes, fats*—and I want to take a little of your time to talk about this. So make yourself a cup of tea, get cozy, and let's dish.

I know that for years, nutrition authorities said that eating fat makes people fat and sick. However, as you know if you're savvy about current research in nutrition, this is not true. In reality, the science shows that *eating the right fats helps you lose fat*—and what's more, eating good fats helps keep you healthy. Here are just some of the most recent findings comparing low-fat diets to diets that include a moderate dose of fat:

- The A TO Z Weight Loss Study lasted twelve months and involved more than three hundred overweight, nondiabetic, premenopausal women. It compared four diets: Atkins (the lowest in carbs and highest in fat), Zone, Ornish, and the LEARN diet.

  The women eating the Atkins diet lost *twice as much weight* as the women eating the other diets—and their cholesterol and blood pressure improved, as well.[23]

- More recently, researchers randomized thirty-four patients with at least two symptoms of metabolic syndrome—a combination of risk factors, including a big belly, high triglycerides, bad cholesterol, high blood pressure, and elevated blood sugar—to a two-week Paleo-style program (which is low in carbs and rich in healthy fats) or a "healthy" calorie-matched diet lower in fat.

  Compared to the low-fat control diet, the Paleo diet resulted in greater reversal of metabolic syndrome symptoms and a greater reduction of cardiovascular risks. What's more, while the goal here was to keep participants' weight unchanged, the researchers say that "more weight loss was observed in the Palaeolithic group."[24]

- Another study compared the effects of a Paleo diet to a standard low-fat diabetic diet on patients with type 2 diabetes.

  Researchers found that compared to the standard diabetes diet, the Paleo diet resulted in lower HbA1c levels (a long-term measure of blood sugar levels), lower triglyceride levels, lower blood pressure levels, and higher levels of HDL ("good") cholesterol. In addition, these dieters lost more weight than the diabetic-diet group.[25]

- Cochrane, a highly respected independent health research group, reviewed low-glycemic and high-glycemic diets. (Low-glycemic diets are rich in fats and low in carbs, while high-glycemic diets are low in fats and high in carbs.)

  The group concluded, "Overweight or obese people on low-glycemic-index diets lost more weight and had more improvement in lipid profiles than those receiving comparison diets. Body mass, total fat mass, body mass index, total cholesterol, and LDL-cholesterol all decreased significantly more in the LGI group."

  What's more, the researchers found that people on the low-glycemic diets did as well as or better than those on calorie-controlled high-glycemic diets *even when the people on the low-glycemic diets were allowed to eat as much as they wanted.*[26]

In short, the facts are in, and the message is clear: A diet that supplies your body with healthy fats will burn more fat off you than a low-fat, high-carb diet. (And since belly fat is the fastest to mobilize, that means your muffin top will go fast.) In addition, the changes in your blood sugar, cholesterol, and triglyceride levels will make your doctor happy!

But, Dr. Kellyann . . . Isn't Saturated Fat Bad for Me?

There's a good chance you already know that avocados, olive oil, nuts, and omega-3-rich fatty fish—foods that doctors put on the "naughty" list not long ago—are now back on the "nice" list. So the idea of adding these foods to your diet may not scare you, especially now that you know that eating fat *burns* fat.

But steaks, burgers, pot roast, and other foods containing saturated fat? Those might give you a fright.

After all, for decades you've heard that eating saturated fat won't just make you fat . . . it'll kill you. Allegedly, eating red meat is the quickest way to drop dead of a stroke or a heart attack. And maybe you saw a recent scare report about coconut oil's high saturated fat content.

But if you're asking, "Dr. Kellyann, do you want me dead?"—no, I most certainly do not! I want you to be showing off a beautiful, slim belly for decades and decades to come. So when I include such foods as red meat and coconut oil on my diet, it's because I know that saturated fat is *not* bad for your cardiovascular system.

If you don't believe it, check out the findings from a 2014 meta-analysis (a powerful type of study that combines data from many other studies). This study found *no* association between saturated fat and all-cause mortality, coronary heart disease, ischemic stroke, or type 2 diabetes. The researchers concluded, "Current evidence does not clearly support cardiovascular guidelines that encourage high consumption of polyunsaturated fatty acids and low consumption of total saturated fats."[27]

Still skittish? Then take a look at a 2015 study in the *British Medical Journal.* This one basically came to the same conclusion: "Saturated fats are not associated with all-cause mortality, cardiovascular disease, coronary heart disease, ischemic stroke, or type 2 diabetes."[28]

As for the coconut oil report, it claimed that this oil might raise levels of LDL ("bad") cholesterol. However, this report was surprisingly out of date when it comes to how we interpret cholesterol levels. We now know that it's not your overall cholesterol but your *ratio of good to bad cholesterol* that matters.

So let's look at the evidence when it comes to coconut oil, cholesterol, and related health markers.

- In one study, forty obese women ate soybean oil or coconut oil three times a day for twelve weeks. They also ate a low-calorie diet and walked fifty minutes a day. Both groups lost weight, but the women eating coconut oil had smaller waist circumferences at the end of the study, while the women eating soybean oil had slightly larger waists. The women eating coconut oil also improved their levels of HDL (the "good" cholesterol) and reduced their levels of C-reactive protein (CRP), a marker of inflammation.[29]

- In another study, researchers asked women to eat a high-fat, coconut oil–based diet; a low-fat, coconut oil–based diet; or a diet containing highly unsaturated fats. The women ate each diet for about three weeks, with a "washout" period in between, during which they ate their typical diets. Women eating the high-fat, coconut oil–based diet significantly lowered their levels of lipoprotein, a blood marker that predicts heart attack risk more accurately than cholesterol levels do.[30]

- Still another study, this one of 116 patients with coronary artery disease, found that a diet rich in coconut oil increased HDL cholesterol (the "good" cholesterol) and decreased waist circumference and body mass.[31]

In short, while coconut oil may raise LDL levels, studies confirm that it also raises HDL levels—and it's the ratio that matters. In addition, the research shows that a diet rich in coconut oil leads to reductions in body mass, a smaller waist circumference, and reductions in markers of inflammations and cardiovascular risk.

So meat won't kill you, and coconut oil won't, either. As cardiologist Aseem Malhotra recently put it, "This idea that dietary saturated fats build up in the coronary arteries is complete unscientific nonsense."[32] I couldn't agree more.

Let me add three cautions here, however:

- First, it does appear that it's not good to eat saturated fat along with huge amounts of carbohydrates and sugar, because this can increase the bad effects of the carbs and sugar. The good news is that on this diet, you'll be slashing the carbs and sugar! If you aren't willing to limit your carb and sugar intake after you finish the diet, then you should limit your saturated fat intake.

- Second, while saturated fats are healthy, you don't want to overload yourself with them. One problem I see in my practice is that many dieters interpret "eat low-carb" to mean "eat tons of fat." That's a bad idea with any fat, no matter how healthy it is. On this diet, you'll eat *small, healthy amounts* of fats.

- Third, different bodies respond in different ways to foods, so the right amount of saturated fat for one person might be too much for another. One thing I stress as a naturopathic physician is to *do what works for your own body*. This may take a little trial and error on your part. For instance, if you aren't taking off weight like crazy, try cutting down a little on your saturated fat (by limiting your intake of red meat or coconut oil, for example), and see what happens.

Simply keep these three rules in mind—especially the one about not overdoing it—and you can eat those saturated fats FEARLESSLY!

What the 10-Day Belly Slimdown Is Going to Do for You—Inside and Out

Right now, I know that your number-one goal is to take off ugly belly fat—and that's my number-one goal for you, too.

However, that's just the *start* of what this diet will do for you! In fact, we're going to *transform* your belly inside and out. I call it the 10-Day Belly Slimdown "two-fer." Over the next ten days, here's what we're going to do:

WE'RE GOING TO SHRINK YOUR BELLY SIZE

On this diet, your excess pounds and inches are going to melt away. That's because we're going to conquer the biggest culprit behind belly fat: excess *insulin*.

As my friend Alan Hopkins, MD, likes to say, insulin is a *"fat fertilizer."* Have you ever seen someone with diabetes go on insulin and then gain twenty to thirty pounds? It happens all the time. Here's a

---

IS THIS DIET RIGHT FOR YOU?

If you want to lose your belly fat, banish your bloat, look and feel younger, and take control over your cravings, you're definitely in the right place. However, here are a few cautions:

First, this is a short-term diet. If you need to diet for longer than ten days to lose the weight you want to lose, use this plan to jump-start your weight loss and then switch to my basic Bone Broth Diet afterward.

If you have any significant medical conditions, or you're taking any medications—especially medications for diabetes—check with your doctor to make sure it's safe for you to do this diet.

If you are diabetic or taking blood sugar–lowering medications, this diet may dramatically lower your blood sugar. That's a very good thing—but your doctor will need to monitor you closely during the diet to make sure you don't become hypoglycemic. DO NOT do this diet unless your diabetes is well controlled.

If you're pregnant or nursing, wait until later to do the diet.

If you're recovering from a significant injury or illness, be sure you're fully healed before starting the diet.

If you have a history of an eating disorder, make sure your doctor gives you the okay to follow this diet.

If you're under eighteen, be sure your mom or dad checks with your doctor before you start the diet.

---

quick explanation of why this phenomenon occurs—and why excess insulin puts weight on your belly even if you aren't diabetic.

When you have too much blood sugar—which virtually *everyone* eating a standard Western diet does—your body keeps cranking out more and more insulin to handle it. This insulin keeps trying to deliver glucose to your cells, even when they don't want it. Eventually, your cells get fed up with this onslaught and respond by slamming the door on insulin and its cargo of glucose. This is the *insulin resistance* I talked about earlier.

When your cells say no to more glucose, insulin ferries it back to your liver and tells the liver to store it in a form called *glycogen*. Once you stockpile more glycogen than you need, your body puts it into long-term storage in (you guessed it) your fat cells. And before long, you need to let that belt out yet another notch.

On this diet, you're not going to eat foods that jack up your insulin levels. Instead, you're going to eat SLIM-gestion foods that will lower your insulin levels and burn fat off you like crazy—up to a pound a day. And you'll ramp up the power of these foods with SLIM-gestion herbs and spices that make the fat fall off even faster.

Want a bonus? At the same time, these SLIM-gestion foods are going to banish your bloat, gas, and constipation. And that will take even *more* inches off your belly.

NOTE: To understand the way insulin is working in your own body, you can order a fasting glucose, a three-month glucose measurement called Hemoglobin A1c, and a fasting insulin. One direct access lab resource we recommend is YourLabWork.com/Dr-Kellyann.

WE'RE GOING TO RAISE YOUR BELLY IQ

Are you sick and tired of constant cravings? On this diet, we're going to get rid of those cravings by resetting your "hunger trigger," making your belly smarter about when it's hungry and when it isn't. This is going to give you total control over your appetite from now on.

How are we going to accomplish this? The answer involves a hormone you might never have heard about: *leptin.*

Leptin is a hormone your fat cells use to communicate with your brain about how much energy you need. High levels of leptin make you feel full, while low levels make you feel hungry. That's why I call leptin your "hunger trigger."

Sounds pretty simple, right? But here's where things can start to go off the rails.

If you eat a standard American diet, which is high in carbohydrates, you can develop *leptin resistance* (which is much like the insulin resistance I just talked about). These foods cause your leptin to spike again and again, all day long, and eventually your brain reacts by tuning it out.

When this happens, your cells don't know that you're full. Instead, they panic because they think you're starving. Even if you don't need food, you suffer deep-down cravings—and you're genetically hard-wired to respond to these cravings by shoveling in high-calorie foods as fast as you can.

Over the next ten days, we're going to make your belly smarter by resetting your leptin "hunger trigger." As a result, you won't crave food unless it's really time to eat . . . and you won't be tempted to stuff yourself with popcorn, pizza, pie, and pasta. We'll also get your body in sync with its natural eating window, so those all-day cravings will vanish.

WE'RE GOING TO LOWER YOUR BELLY AGE

These days, one of the hottest topics is the *microbiome*—the entire ecosystem of microbes inside the gut. That's because the microbiome is a key player in everything from immune function to mood to weight.

Now, here's something you need to know: If you have a big belly, it's a virtual *guarantee* that you have a sick microbiome. And to get rid of that belly fat, you need to heal your microbiome.

In fact, one of the biggest reasons for the current obesity epidemic in this country is that we have another epidemic: an epidemic of sick guts. That's because most of us eat inflammatory foods, take medications (such as antibiotics and NSAIDs) that whack gut bugs, get too little exercise, and deal with too much stress. All these things sicken good gut bugs while letting bad bugs gain a foothold.

If this happens to you, your gut will become inflamed. (Think of

ANGIE

Angie, a professional dancer and a patient of mine, never had trouble controlling her weight. Then she hit twenty-eight—which is approaching ancient in her career—and things changed.

Don't get me wrong. Angie still looked gorgeous. But while *gorgeous* is good enough for most people, it isn't for a career dancer. A professional dancer needs to look absolutely, utterly perfect. (Have you ever watched the pros on *Dancing with the Stars*? Do you see an extra ounce on any of them?) And perfection is especially critical for dancers who are edging toward thirty and facing competition from flawless twenty-year-olds.

Angie was about one inch of belly fat away from having to find a new career. To add to her stress, she had an audition for a life-changing role in just two weeks. When she came to me, she was in a panic.

I put Angie on my diet. She followed it religiously—which didn't surprise me, since she had so much at stake.

Angie lost the weight. We trimmed that waist down. She looked amazing when she went for her audition. And she got the job.

this like a sunburn, only on the inside.) This inflammation, in turn, will damage the walls of your intestines—and that's when things *really* go bad.

When your gut wall weakens, little holes open up in it. We call this *intestinal permeability*, or a "leaky gut." A leaky gut lets toxins and undigested food molecules escape from your intestines, and they wind up on the wrong side of your gut wall.

Your immune system immediately spots these invaders and sounds an alarm. Then it goes on the attack, releasing a flood of invader-fighting chemicals. Unfortunately, these chemicals wind up poisoning your own cells in a classic case of "friendly fire." The result: sick, inflamed cells.

FIVE KEYS TO BUSTING BELLY FAT

ALAN HOPKINS, MD

Metabolism and Weight Loss Expert, Clinical Assistant Professor
of Surgery and Perioperative Care, Dell Medical School,
University of Texas at Austin

We used to think our belly fat was only a place where we stored excess energy, but it turns out it is one of the most significant hormone factories of the body. If these hormones get out of balance, they can lead to chronic inflammation, dyslipidemia (abnormal lipids in the blood), early heart disease, and diabetes. Measuring these hormones can give us an idea of the health of our belly fat—and don't be fooled, there are skinny people out there who have sick belly fat, too.

Genetically, we all have different abilities to recruit new fat cells when we need them. If we can't make new fat cells fast enough, our existing fat cells swell and get sick, releasing hormones that have far-reaching effects on our bodies.

The five things you can do to improve the health of your belly fat now are:

1. Reduce processed sugar intake to less than 25 grams per day to reduce insulin levels. (The average American eats 150 to 200 grams of processed sugar per day.) Remember that excess insulin is a "fat fertilizer."

2. Get at least 7.5 hours of sleep per day, since we principally burn our belly fat during deep sleep.

3. Exercise (high-intensity training is best), keeping in mind that resistance training will also recruit new muscle cells, which will also help lower insulin.

4. Reduce your stress to improve the function of cortisol, another fat-fertilizing hormone.

5. Consider advanced biomarker testing to evaluate the health of your belly fat. You can measure your "good" and "bad" fat

hormones. The good fat hormone is called adiponectin and is cardio-protective at higher levels. Low levels are associated with a dramatic risk for diabetes and coronary artery disease.[33, 34] Leptin is the "bad" fat hormone when it's elevated, because it's pro-inflammatory and is associated with early aging of the cardiovascular system. A resource for you to directly access lab testing for these hormones is YourLabWork .com/Dr-Kellyann.

Over time, as your leaky gut keeps letting toxins escape, your immune system gets stuck in the "on" position. As a result, inflammation spreads throughout your entire body—like a forest fire that never goes out. This inflammation screws up your hormones, wrecks your metabolism, and makes you fat and sick inside.

We now know that this inflammation is the *root cause of obesity*. We also know that we need to battle it at ground zero: the gut. To do that, we need to feed your gut the foods it craves—and get rid of the foods that are sickening and aging it.

On this diet, we're going to do just that. As a result, we'll lower the inflammation in your gut, which in turn will reduce inflammation throughout your entire body—and that's going to slash your belly fat. In addition, it's going to cut your risk for diseases of aging, such as diabetes, heart disease, and cancer.

Now let's talk about two more big benefits you'll get from this diet—benefits that go beyond shrinking, healing, and "wising up" your belly. Here they are:

WE'RE GOING TO LOAD YOUR BELLY WITH BODY-BEAUTIFYING COLLAGEN

Every day on this diet, you'll feed your gut collagen-rich shakes and bone broth. Your gut won't just use this collagen to heal itself; it'll also mainline it to your skin, hair, and nails, where it's going to smooth those wrinkles, restore your hair's beautiful bounce, and make your nails strong and healthy again.

WE'RE GOING TO LOAD YOUR BELLY
WITH JOINT-HEALING NUTRIENTS

Do you find that activities you did easily a decade ago—jogging, climbing stairs, lifting boxes—now lead to aches and pains? That's because you're suffering from damage to the cartilage in your joints.

The bone broth you'll drink on this diet is brimming with glucosamine and chondroitin—the same nutrients many doctors prescribe to make your joints limber and pain-free again. These healing nutrients will travel from your gut to all the joints in your body, soothing and rejuvenating them.

My Triple-Punch . . . and More!

Now you know our plan for the next ten days. We're going to slash belly fat off you by:

- Shrinking your eating window to make your fat burning soar

- Loading you with bone broth—my "liquid gold"

- Filling you up with collagen and other fat-melting SLIM-gestion superfoods to take your metabolism to new heights

As a result, you'll lose up to a pound a day and take inches off your waist. We're also going to banish your bloat, take years or even decades off your "inner belly," tame your cravings, and—as a bonus—give you gorgeous skin, strong hair and nails, and happier joints.

How's that for amazing? I know you signed on for the weight loss . . . but there's so, *so* much more that this diet will do for you. I'm not kidding when I say that it will change your life.

And guess what: We're not going to transform your body through diet alone. That's because I have three more tricks up my sleeve! Here's what we're going to do in addition:

- We're going to slim and sculpt your abs with exercises that will start to firm up that "pooch" within weeks.

- We're going to lower your levels of *cortisol*, because this stress hormone is another reason you have that belly.

- We're going to cleanse your insides from head to toe, sweeping out the toxins that make you sick, pack pounds onto your middle, and age your inner belly.

And you know what? I'm not done yet!

Once you finish your diet, I'm going to tell you how to keep that slim belly for the rest of your life. On my Slim Belly Forever plan, you'll eat three meals of *delicious* food every day. What's more, you won't need to give up *any* food you truly love. (You can even have an occasional doughnut—I promise.) And you'll never, ever, *ever* need to diet again.

That's my 10-Day Belly Slimdown approach. It's fast. It's powerful. It works for my clinical patients, and it works for my celebrity clients. It works not just for now, but for life. And it will work for you.

So here's my question: Are you ready to lose your belly fat fast . . . and keep it off forever?

Then let's *do* it.

MY 10-DAY DIET TO *CRUSH* YOUR BELLY FAT

Okay, let's get down to it.

How committed are you? Do you want to get that belly fat off *right now*, and are you willing to do what it takes?

Then it's time for me to introduce you to the diet that will make it vanish—*poof*. This same diet is going to eliminate your bloat, heal your inner belly, and cut your cravings down to size.

But first, let me spell out the rules. For the next ten days, you're going to eat the foods on the 10-Day Belly Slimdown "yes" list—and *only* these foods. If a food isn't on the list, don't eat it. Only eat *as much* as I tell you to eat, and—most important of all—only eat *when* I tell you to eat. Period. No cheating. No sneaking snacks. No second helpings. No eating outside of your eating window. No exceptions.

If I sound like an army drill sergeant, that's intentional. I'm usually a huggy, softhearted little teddy bear, but *not* when it comes to stripping off belly fat in a hurry. That's because the magic only happens if you commit 100%. Not 70%. Not 80%. Not 90%.

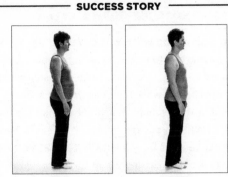

BEFORE   AFTER

GAIL PEREZ

WEIGHT LOST: 6.2 POUNDS | BELLY INCHES LOST: 6.5

Gail says that as a result of her ten-day diet, "I have a lot of energy. I don't feel sleepy in the middle of the afternoon. I also don't feel that crash like I need to eat immediately or I'm going to pass out. . . . I just feel better overall and have noticed my clothes feel looser."

She did need to tough her way through the "carb flu" and battled symptoms including headaches. However, she says, "After a couple days it went away, as did the hunger pains."

So if you're tempted to cheat, picture my face right in your face and hear me yelling, *"PUT THE MARGARITA DOWN—NOW!"*

Here's the bottom line. If you want insane results in ten days, then you need to follow this program to the letter. If you cheat, that's fine—nobody's perfect—but you'll need to *start all over again,* from Day 1.

Are you willing to accept my tough terms for ten days in order to get the sexy abs you're craving—those same spectacular abs I put on New York and Hollywood celebrities? Are you willing to white-knuckle it in order to lose the weight, banish the bloat, and—as a bonus—get happy joints and gorgeous skin, hair, and nails?

Then get your game face on—because here we go.

My 10-Day Slimdown Program

Each day of your diet has four phases. Here's an overview of all four phases, followed by an At-a-Glance chart to make following the diet simple.

PHASE 1: "BROTH BURNING"—FROM WAKE-UP TIME TILL NOON

THIS IS WHERE YOU'LL REALLY BLAST THAT BELLY FAT!

During this phase, you'll have NOTHING but broth—as little as one 8-ounce mug and up to six mugs—along with the beverages I list on page 41. For extra fat-burning and insulin-lowering power, you can add herbs and spices to your broth—see the list on pages 49–51.

While you're waiting for "go time"—the start of your eating window—you can also drink:

- Unsweetened black coffee (an excellent appetite suppressant)—including my Collagen Coffee, which gives you an extra burst of collagen power to slim you down and quell your cravings

- Unsweetened black, white, green, or herbal tea

- Water with half a lemon or less squeezed into it (to help detoxify your body)

Do not use artificial sweeteners during the "broth burning" period. Also, don't add any dairy or nondairy creamers (milk, almond milk, coconut milk, etc.) to your coffee or tea.

Remember: just broth, coffee, Collagen Coffee, tea, and lemon water—*nothing else*. This will extend your fasting window so you burn fat like *mad*.

BONE BROTH BUYING TIPS

If you want to make your own bone broth, it's super simple. You'll find lots of basic recipes and fun variations in the recipe section, along with tips for getting the best results.

But if you're too busy to make your own broth, that's no problem! These days, many health food stores carry bone broth, and you can also order it online. Just follow these two rules:

- Buy organic broth that's specifically labeled "bone broth"—not just broth.

- Read labels carefully and make sure your broth is *only* bone broth with natural vegetables, herbs, and spices and doesn't contain other ingredients such as yeast extract, molasses, corn syrup, or cane sugar. My Bone Broth, which you can order online, is a great option.

For times when heating liquid broth isn't convenient, you can use Dr. Kellyann's Powdered Bone Broth packets anywhere. (This is a great solution if you're traveling.) Simply mix with hot water, and you're good to go!

PHASE 2: A SLIMMING SHAKE—
BETWEEN NOON AND 1:00 P.M.

NOW IT'S TIME FOR A DOSE OF THAT FAT-NUKING, WRINKLE-BLASTING COLLAGEN!

Your first meal of the day will be a hearty, delicious shake that will fill you up and load you with fiber. Your shake will include:

- A high-quality protein powder or collagen powder

- Two handfuls of non-starchy vegetables from the list on page 47

WHAT PROTEIN OR COLLAGEN POWDER SHOULD YOU USE?

At the grocery or health food store, you'll see rows and rows of protein powders. Here are three simple rules for choosing the right one:

- If you opt for beef protein or collagen powder, select a high-quality product made from pastured beef. Be sure to look specifically for the word *beef* on the label. My protein powders are a great choice; you can find them at DrKellyann.com.

- If you're choosing a whey protein, make sure you buy *whey protein isolate* rather than *whey protein concentrate.* Many people are sensitive to the lactose in whey protein, but whey protein isolate is lactose-free. (For more on this, see "Say Yes to Whey!" on page 126.) Be sure to look for the word *isolate* on the label.

- Choose pea protein only if you're doing the vegetarian version of the diet (see page 56). Pea protein is higher in carbs and isn't as nutrient-dense as beef or whey protein.

One serving of protein or collagen powder is equal to one to two scoops of powder. Plan to have 15 to 25 grams of protein in each shake.

- One portion of healthy fat from the list on page 48

- A handful of blueberries if you want extra sweetness

- Herbs and spices for flavor and fat-burning power (see pages 49–51)

- Stevia or monk fruit sweetener, if you like

PHASE 3: "BROTH LOADING"—AFTERNOON AND EVENING TILL 6:00 OR 7:00 P.M.

THIS WILL SATISFY YOUR CRAVINGS, DETOX YOUR BODY, AND LOAD YOU WITH BLOAT-BUSTING FIBER.

In this phase, you'll load up on broth—as little as one 8-ounce mug and up to six mugs.

This time, your broth will also include:

- Two handfuls of chopped leafy green vegetables or other non-starchy veggies per mug. You need the fiber in those veggies to help keep things moving and blast that bloat!

- A little dose of healthy fat (optional)

You can simply toss your chopped greens into your broth, or you can have fun with the "broth loading" soup recipes in Chapter 5.

PHASE 4: A "SLIM PLATE" MEAL— BETWEEN 6:00 AND 7:00 P.M.

TIME FOR MORE OF THOSE HIGH-OCTANE SLIM-GESTION FOODS!

Your last meal of the day will be a SLIM Plate meal including protein, vegetables, herbs, and spices, along with a serving of fat to help fill you up. You'll also add the fat-burning power of grapefruit (see note below) or berries. For great SLIM Plate ideas, see Chapter 8.

NOTE: If you are taking any medications, check with your doctor before adding grapefruit to your diet. Grapefruit and grapefruit juice interact with many medications (for instance, statins), significantly

YOUR SLIM PLATE PORTION GUIDE

PROTEIN PORTIONS

A serving of meat, fish, or poultry should be about the size and thickness of your palm. A serving of eggs is as many as you can hold in your hand (that's two or three for women, three or four for men). A serving of egg whites alone is double the serving for whole eggs. Each meal should include a serving of protein.

Note: Don't skimp on your protein! In fact, if you desire, you can increase your protein portion by half. The more we're learning about protein, the more we're finding that people—especially women—need plenty of it to stay young, strong, and healthy.

NON-STARCHY VEGETABLE PORTIONS

A serving of vegetables should be at least the size of a softball. Fill your plate with at least two or three softballs' worth, and add at least two handfuls to each shake. Toss them into your afternoon broth, too!

BERRIES OR GRAPEFRUIT

A serving of fruit is 1/2 a grapefruit or a closed handful of berries.

FAT PORTIONS

A serving of oil or clarified butter is 1 tablespoon.

A serving of nuts, coconut flakes, or olives is about one closed handful.

A serving of nut butter is 1 tablespoon.

A serving of avocado is 1/4 to 1/2 an avocado.

A serving of full-fat coconut milk is 1/3 to 1/2 the can.

A serving of chia seeds is 4 teaspoons.

A serving of flaxseed is 2 tablespoons.

A serving of hemp seeds is 2 tablespoons.

increasing their effects (not a good thing, as it can lead to toxic side effects). If you are taking a medication that interacts with grapefruit, simply add berries to your meal instead.

Here are a few guidelines for your SLIM Plates:

- Your protein should be free from nitrates, nitrites, gluten, sugar, and artificial colors and flavors. For a list of approved proteins, see page 47.

- Your meal must contain one serving of healthy fat. For a list of approved fats, see page 48.

- You can load your plate with non-starchy veggies. Use approved veggies from the list on page 47.

- For extra gut-healing power, include probiotic foods such as fresh sauerkraut, fresh pickles, and kimchi (for more on these foods, see page 142).

- After you finish this meal, you'll have nothing else to eat or drink for the rest of the day except tea, coffee, water, or bone broth.

When you're making your evening meal, you don't need to weigh your food or count calories, carbs, or fat grams. Simply follow these rules, and you can't go wrong!

Your Daily Diet at a Glance

Still sorting out the four phases of your 10-Day Belly Slimdown? The chart on page 46 will help you visualize your plan easily.

I recommend flagging that page so you can reference it easily. Better yet, print out the "Your Daily Diet at a Glance" chart on the Resources page on my website, drkellyann.com/gift, and stick it on your fridge. That way, you'll know exactly what to do all day long.

SLIM-gestion "Yes" Foods

To make it easy for you to know what to eat (and what to avoid) on this diet, there's a quick list of the "yes" foods starting on page 47. Keep this handy, and take a copy of it with you when you go shopping. You'll also find a printable list of these foods on the Resources page on my website, drkellyann.com/gift.

YOUR DAILY DIET AT A GLANCE

PHASE 1	PHASE 2	PHASE 3	PHASE 4
MORNING "BROTH BURNING" (from wake-up to noon*)	AFTERNOON SHAKE (noon–1:00 p.m.*)	AFTERNOON "BROTH LOADING" (between your shake and evening meal)	SLIM PLATE MEAL (6:00–7:00 p.m.*)
* You can adjust your shake and evening meal times to suit your schedule; just make sure to eat your meals within a seven-hour window.			
Broth with herbs and spices (up to six 8-ounce cups) Unsweetened coffee, Collagen Coffee, or tea—no dairy or nondairy creamer Lemon water or plain water	1 to 2 scoops protein or collagen powder (15 to 25 grams) 2 handfuls of non-starchy veggies 1 serving of fat from list of approved fats **Optional:** Dr. Kellyann's Collagen Coffee for more collagen power! **Optional:** 1 closed handful of blueberries **Optional:** Stevia or monk fruit sweetener Water or ice	Bone broth with herbs, spices, and 2 handfuls of non-starchy veggies in each mug (up to six 8-ounce cups) **OR** Soups made with bone broth (be sure to follow the recipes in Chapter 4—these are specifically designed for the diet) **OR** Plain bone broth plus a side salad of greens sprinkled with lemon juice or up to 1 tablespoon vinaigrette Water, lemon water, coffee, Collagen Coffee, or tea **Optional:** Stevia or monk fruit sweetener in your beverages	1 serving of protein 1 serving of approved fat Unlimited non-starchy vegetables ½ grapefruit or 1 handful of berries Tea, coffee, Collagen Coffee, lemon water, or bone broth

APPROVED PROTEINS

COLLAGEN OR PROTEIN POWDER

BEEF

CHICKEN

LAMB

TURKEY

WILD BOAR

PORK (pastured only)

FISH (be sure canned fish is packed in olive oil or water)

EGGS

ORGAN MEATS

NITRITE-, NITRATE-, AND GLUTEN-FREE DELI MEATS (read labels carefully and make sure you're not getting any sugars or artificial additives)

NOTE: If you can afford it, buy pastured meat, chicken, and eggs. These are cleaner than factory-farmed meat, and they're much higher in fat-burning nutrients. However, if your budget is tight, regular meat is just fine. Simply cut the fat off meat and take the skin off chicken, because that's where most of the toxins are. Avoid pork unless you can find pastured pork; luckily, more and more stores are carrying pastured pork these days.

APPROVED VEGETABLES

You can add any veggies from this list to your shakes, afternoon broth, and evening meal:

ARUGULA

ASPARAGUS

BELL PEPPERS

BOK CHOY

BROCCOLI

BROCCOLI RABE

BRUSSELS SPROUTS

CAULIFLOWER

CELERY

CHILE PEPPERS

CILANTRO

CUCUMBERS

DAIKON

EGGPLANT

GARLIC

GREEN BEANS

GREEN CABBAGE

GREEN ONIONS

GREENS (beet,collard, mustard, and turnip greens)

JALAPEÑO PEPPERS

KALE

KONJAC ROOT (SHIRATAKI)

LEEKS

LETTUCE

MUSHROOMS

NAPA CABBAGE

ONIONS

PARSLEY

RADICCHIO

RADISHES

RED CABBAGE

SEAWEED

SPINACH

SPROUTS

SUMMER SQUASH

SWISS CHARD

TOMATO

WATERCRESS

ZUCCHINI

DO NOT EAT starchy vegetables (potatoes, sweet potatoes, yams, pumpkin, carrots, butternut squash, spaghetti squash, beets, turnips, parsnips, plantains, green peas, corn, or taro).

If possible, add a daily serving of a probiotic food such as fresh sauerkraut or kimchi, and include prebiotic veggies such as asparagus and onions. (For more on the power of probiotics and prebiotics, see page 142).

APPROVED FATS

Choose one serving of fat from this list for your shake, your afternoon broth loading phase (fat is optional in that phase), and your evening meal:

COCONUT OIL / MCT OIL
(1 tablespoon per serving)

OLIVE OIL (1 tablespoon per serving)

AVOCADO OIL (1 tablespoon per serving)

WALNUT OIL (1 tablespoon per serving)

GHEE (clarified butter, with the milk solids removed; page 147; 1 tablespoon per serving)

CANNED FULL-FAT COCONUT MILK ($1/3$ to $1/2$ [14-ounce] can)

COCONUT CHIPS (unsweetened; 1 closed handful or about 2 tablespoons per serving)

AVOCADO ($1/4$ to $1/2$ avocado per serving)

OLIVES (1 closed handful per serving or about 2 tablespoons)

ALMOND BUTTER (unsweetened; 1 tablespoon per serving)

NUTS (1 closed handful per serving, about 2 tablespoons)

CHIA SEEDS (4 teaspoons per serving)

HEMP SEEDS (2 tablespoons per serving)

GROUND FLAXSEED (2 tablespoons per serving)

POWER UP YOUR FAT-BURNING WITH SLIM-GESTION HERBS AND SPICES!

On this diet, you're going to load your body with weight-loss superfoods. And believe it or not, some of the most powerful fat-burning nutrients come in the smallest packages: the dried herbs and spices in your pantry and the fresh herbs in your garden.

You already love these seasonings because they make your meals taste great. But right now, I want you to use them for another reason: They'll help you *blast* your belly fat. This is why I want you to flavor your morning and afternoon broth—as well as your shakes and SLIM Plate meals—with as many of them as you can.

In particular, the following herbs and spices can ramp up your fat burning—so go crazy with them!

- Basil—Basil is anti-inflammatory, reduces water retention and bloating, and functions as an *adaptogen* (a substance that helps your body adapt to stress). Basil also helps reduce fat buildup in your liver while detoxifying your body.

- Black pepper—*Piperine* is the compound that gives pepper its pungent flavor. Piperine enhances the effects of curcumin, the active ingredient in turmeric—a fat-burning powerhouse I'll talk about later. One study also suggests that the piperine in black pepper battles fat formation.[1]

- Cardamom—Cardamom is *thermogenic* (meaning it increases your body heat and speeds up your metabolism), has anti-inflammatory properties, and acts as an antioxidant, cleaning up rogue molecules called free radicals and resisting cellular aging.

- Cayenne—*Capsaicin*, the compound that gives chile peppers their heat, helps shrink fatty tissue and lower blood-fat levels. It's also thermogenic.

- Cilantro and coriander—Although both names refer to the same plant, *cilantro* typically refers to the leafy green part of the coriander plant, while *coriander* is the common name for the seeds of the plant. Both cilantro and coriander are antioxidant-rich and may help reduce LDL, or "bad," cholesterol levels in your blood. They also contain large quantities of vitamins A and K.

- Cinnamon—Cinnamon helps regulate blood glucose levels, reducing your cravings and helping you burn fat faster.

- Cloves—Cloves help reduce your blood sugar. They also help improve your digestion and optimize your metabolism.

- Cumin—Cumin is a great fat burner that also aids in digestion. One teaspoon can help you burn up to three times more body fat!

- Fennel seeds—These are a natural diuretic and a powerful digestive aid.

- Garlic—Garlic helps burn belly fat. It also reduces LDL cholesterol, which may lower your risk of heart disease. In addition, it reduces oxidative damage from free radicals, helping fight the aging process.

- Ginger—Ginger has anti-inflammatory properties, and it's a powerful gut soother. It also has thermogenic properties that help boost your metabolism.

- Green tea—Green tea is loaded with antioxidants and thermogenic properties. What's more, the EGCG in green tea reduces the amount of fat your body absorbs when you eat.

- Mustard—One teaspoon of prepared mustard can boost your metabolism by up to 25% for several hours after eating. The credit goes to allyl isothiocyanates, which are phytochemicals that give mustard its characteristic flavor.

- Parsley—Parsley's wealth of vitamin C makes it a great immune-system booster. It's also an excellent source of beta-carotene, an antioxidant that helps protect your body against free-radical damage. It has anti-inflammatory properties, relaxes your muscles, and encourages digestion.

- Turmeric—Curcumin is the active ingredient in turmeric. It slows the formation of fatty tissue by affecting the blood vessels needed to form it. Curcumin contributes to lower body fat and weight loss. It is also an anti-inflammatory agent and lowers insulin resistance.

- White pepper—Just as in black pepper, piperine is the compound that gives white pepper its pungent flavor. Like black pepper, white pepper increases the effects of curcumin, the active ingredient in turmeric.

As you can see, those little herbs and spices have incredible mojo. (It's true: Good things do come in small packages!) So use a liberal hand when you add them to your meals, put them in your shakes, or stir them into your broth.

FOUR STEPS TO TAKE BEFORE YOU START YOUR DIET

I hope that you're really jazzed about getting that belly fat off your body. If that's the case, I know you may want to start right now.

However, the way to ace this diet is to go into it fully prepared. Before you dive in, I want you to lay a little groundwork. Here are four things I want you to do before Day 1.

1. COLLECT YOUR STARTING-LINE STATS.

To see how far you've come at the end of this diet, you need to know where you started out. So write down the number on your bathroom scale. Then measure your belly circumference with a measuring tape, positioning the tape over your belly button.

If you don't have a measuring tape, no worries—just use a piece of yarn or string, cutting it to the size of your waist. When you're done, you can wrap the yarn around your waist again, mark the new measurement with a pen, and then measure the difference with a ruler.

If you're *really* into keeping score, you can also calculate your waist-to-hip ratio, which is more important than your belly measurement alone when it comes to health risks. Women with a waist-to-hip ratio greater than 0.8, and men with a ratio greater than 1.0, are at increased risk for health problems because of the way their fat is distributed. To calculate your waist-to-hip ratio, start with your waist measurement. Then measure your hips, putting the tape over the biggest part of your butt. Finally, divide your waist measurement by your hip measurement.

There are also biometric scales that can measure total body fat percentage, muscle percentage, and visceral fat percentage. If you want more data to motivate you, buying a scale like this might be a great idea.

If your doctor says you have metabolic syndrome or "prediabetes," or you have a diagnosis of diabetes, I also want you to note what your blood sugar levels are at the start and end of your diet. In addition, you might want to list your starting cholesterol levels and blood pressure.

Finally, take some "selfies"—front-view and profile—wearing a bikini or shorts and a sports bra. After you finish your diet, you can take a new set of selfies and celebrate the difference.

To help you chart your progress, you'll find a Measurement Tracker on page 268, and there's also a copy on the Resources page on my website at drkellyann.com/gift.

2. GET RID OF "NO" FOODS.

The best way to avoid taboo foods is to get them out of your house. So before you begin your diet, ask a friend to store any foods that aren't allowed, as well as any alcohol.

When you clean out your "no" foods, be *thorough*. Right now, you might not be tempted by that year-old Fudgsicle stuck to the bottom of your freezer. But on Day 5 of your diet, when the "carb flu" strikes (see page 71), it might look absolutely *awesome*. Remember: You can't eat it if it's not there!

3. PREP THE FOODS FOR YOUR 10-DAY BELLY SLIMDOWN.

You're going to be eating real food all day on this diet. And if you're used to microwaved frozen meals or dinner from a can, I know this will be a big change.

But not to worry! There are two ways to prepare for your diet. One is to spend an hour or so in the store or online buying high-quality ready-to-go foods. In this approach, you hardly need to cook at all. The other is to spend a few hours in the kitchen before you start your diet, prepping the foods you'll need. (This is called "batch prep," and people who are into healthy eating are crazy about it. You'll find tons of tips on it on Pinterest and in fitness and nutrition blogs.)

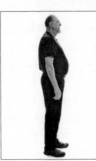 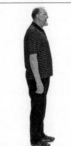

BEFORE   AFTER

LARRY McCAMMON

WEIGHT LOST: 9 POUNDS | BELLY INCHES LOST: 4

You'd think that losing nine pounds and four inches of belly fat would thrill Larry more than anything—but he's even more excited about the changes in his blood sugar.

"I had been on insulin for a couple of years now, and I had steadily increased it," he says. "I haven't taken any for eleven days. I was taking 25 units of long-acting insulin in the morning and at night and 16 units of regular insulin in the morning and at night. It's wonderful to look at my [blood] sugar and not worry about it, and it's been wonderful to not have to take shots twice a day."

In addition, he's pleased that his skin looks better, and he reports one more change: the hair in his mustache now looks less gray!

Hearing this doesn't surprise me, because I keep hearing similar comments from people who say their hair is less gray after doing the 10-Day Belly Slimdown or the Bone Broth Diet. Right now, it's all anecdotal . . . but this just may be another surprising benefit of my "liquid gold."

Either way, this is your *up-front investment in total success.* Before you start your diet, turn to Chapter 4 and see how easy it is to fill your fridge, pantry, and freezer ahead of time with ready-to-go or easy-to-assemble meals.

4. VISUALIZE YOUR GOALS.

Before you start your diet, I want you to think hard about your reasons for doing it. This is a big deal, because getting your goals firmly in mind will keep you laser-focused when you otherwise might be tempted to stray.

So ask yourself right now: *What will I get for all my hard work?*

Maybe you want to wear a sexy swimsuit at the beach this year. Maybe you want to lose weight fast before a party or a class reunion. Or maybe you have a family history of cancer, diabetes, or other health problems related to excess belly fat, and you want to slash your own risk.

Whatever your goals are, I want you to *write them down*. In fact, I recommend taping your list to your bathroom mirror where you'll see it every day.

Over the course of your 10-Day Belly Slimdown, there will be times when a doughnut or a slice of pizza sings its siren song to you. But when you keep your eyes on the prize, you'll remain strong and stay the course.

And believe me: At the end of those ten days, you'll *love* yourself for following through and making those big goals a reality!

P.S. Want to be part of a supportive community that will cheer you on? Join our private Facebook group at facebook.com/drkellyann.

FAQs

Over the years, I've helped lots and lots of people lose weight on this diet—and in that time, I've heard several questions over and over again. Here they are:

MAY I STAY ON THIS DIET FOR MORE THAN TEN DAYS?

If you haven't lost all the weight you want to lose at the end of ten days, I recommend switching to my 21-Day Bone Broth Diet. My 10-Day Belly Slimdown is designed to jump-start weight loss, while the Bone Broth Diet is a diet you can stay on as long as necessary.

If you switch to the Bone Broth Diet, you'll alternate a diet of slimming foods with two days of bone broth "mini-fasts" per week—an approach that science shows is ideal for long-term weight loss and anti-aging benefits.

MAY I ALTER THE ROTATION—FOR INSTANCE, BY REPLACING MY EVENING MEAL WITH A SECOND SHAKE?

You can if there's a good reason for it, but you'll get the best results if you stick to one shake and one SLIM Plate meal. That's because you'll get the widest possible range of fat-blasting nutrients.

MAY I SKIP A MEAL?

Yes, but I don't recommend it. If you get hungry, you'll be more tempted to cheat. Trust me: You can eat all the food on this diet and still lose belly fat like crazy!

MAY I SUBSTITUTE REGULAR BROTH FOR BONE BROTH?

No. If you do, your results won't be as good, because you won't get the gut-healing, fat-burning nutrients that bone broth offers. If you don't have time to make your own bone broth, you can find it in many health food stores or order it online at DrKellyann.com.

I KNOW I'LL PROBABLY LOSE A LOT OF WEIGHT QUICKLY ON THIS DIET. BUT ISN'T IT BETTER TO LOSE WEIGHT SLOWLY AND GRADUALLY?

A study by researchers at the University of Florida tackled this very question. The researchers divided 262 women into three groups (fast, moderate, and slow) based on how much weight they lost at the beginning of a diet. They found that women with the fastest weight loss during the first four weeks of dieting had lost significantly more weight by the six-month mark than those who lost weight at a moderate or slow rate at the outset. The rapid weight-losers also maintained a significantly greater weight loss at the eighteen-month mark than the slow group did. And finally, compared to the other groups, the women in the quick-weight-loss group did *not* gain back more weight after their diets ended. So achieving a big weight loss quickly is a smart diet strategy![2]

CAN I DO THIS DIET IF I'M A VEGETARIAN?

Yes, you can! In fact, I've helped hundreds of vegetarians lose weight on a modified version of this diet. (Trust me: You don't work with Hollywood celebs without having a vegetarian option up your sleeve.)

It's true that you may not lose quite as much weight or as many inches as you would on the standard plan. However, you'll still blast a *lot* of belly fat.

Here's how to turn this into a vegetarian diet. (Important: Follow these guidelines ONLY if you are doing the vegetarian diet!) First, substitute a rich vegetable broth (there's a recipe on my website) for the bone broth. If you're a pescetarian, you can substitute fish broth instead (you'll find a recipe in Chapter 4). Next, substitute pea or hemp protein for the beef protein powder in your shake.

Eggs are a great protein choice for your evening meal. In addition, you can stretch the basic diet template—again, ONLY if you are a vegetarian!—to include beans and lentils, edamame, full-fat pastured-milk kefir and yogurt, natto, and tempeh.

However, do avoid veggie chicken wings, soy milk, tofu hot dogs, and related foods. I call these "Frankenfoods" because they're loaded with unhealthy ingredients.

WILL I GET ENOUGH NUTRIENTS ON THIS DIET?

The majority of Americans are nutrient deficient. My diet, in contrast, is going to provide you with tons of micronutrients to keep your metabolism in hyperdrive.

If you're concerned, however, feel free to take a multivitamin and multimineral supplement or any other supplements you currently take; just be sure to take any supplements with a meal.

Also, consider taking these supplements:

BRANCHED-CHAIN AMINO ACIDS

These amino acids help you maintain lean muscle mass as you lose weight.

OMEGA-3 FATTY ACIDS

These fatty acids form the outer lining of your cells. Omega-3 fatty acids decrease inflammation, increase HDL (good cholesterol), lower triglycerides, and change "bad" (LDL) cholesterol into the more favorable type of cholesterol.

VITAMIN D

Vitamin D is more than just a vitamin; it's actually a hormone and is important for every cell in your body. Studies show that vitamin D can help insulin work more efficiently.

COQ10

CoQ10 is a potent antioxidant and plays a key role in energy production in every cell in your body. CoQ10 also boosts heart health and stimulates the production of insulin in your pancreas. The amount of CoQ10 in your body naturally declines with age, making it especially important to supplement after age fifty or if you're on medications that can cause its depletion (such as statin drugs).

Direct access lab testing with YourLabWork.com/Dr-Kellyann can provide baseline measurements of these important nutrients that are essential for optimal metabolism.

ISN'T IT BAD FOR MY CHOLESTEROL TO EAT AS MANY EGGS AS YOU ALLOW ON THIS DIET?

No. It's true that eggs are high in cholesterol, which is why health authorities used to tell you to limit yourself to one or two a week. We now know, however, that when you eat eggs, your liver compensates by producing less cholesterol. As a result, your cholesterol hardly changes at all. That's why a draft of the new Dietary Guidelines for America states, "Cholesterol is not a nutrient of concern for overconsumption."[3]

So go ahead and eat that omelet without fear. In addition to being harmless when it comes to your cholesterol, eggs are loaded with choline—one of nature's most potent fat-blasters.

I'M DOING OKAY WITHOUT SWEETS, BUT I'M REALLY CRAVING DAIRY FOODS. IS THAT NORMAL?

Yes. Dairy products contain opioid peptides similar to the endorphins your body manufactures to make you feel good. These chemicals are addictive, which can make it a bit of a challenge for you to give up your dairy habit. Hang in there, and your cravings for milk and cheese will pass.

WHY CAN'T I USE ARTIFICIAL SWEETENERS?

I know that diet soda seems like a gift from the gods, because you get all the sweetness with none of the guilt. But like most things that seem too good to be true—for instance, your last date's online profile—it is. In fact, there's a chance that diet drinks are as bad for your health and your belly as sugar is.

In one recent study, for instance, researchers asked seven lean, healthy people who weren't diet soda drinkers to consume the maximum acceptable daily dose of artificial sweeteners every day for a single week. Four of the volunteers developed blood sugar problems, because the artificial sweeteners messed with their gut bacteria in a way that led to glucose intolerance.[4]

This means that diet soft drinks are doing the *opposite* of what they should do. Instead of helping you get thin, they're making you fat—because glucose intolerance makes you hungry, tempting you to eat more than you should, and makes it harder for you to burn fat, as well. So even when you're done with this diet, try to break that artificial sweetener habit.

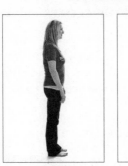

BEFORE   AFTER

KELLY GARBACIK

WEIGHT LOST: 4.6 POUNDS | BELLY INCHES LOST: 2.75

Kelly started out just a few pounds short of her goal weight, so her results are fantastic. (We all know how hard it is to lose those last few pounds!)

As a result of the diet, she says, "I have so much more energy. I love the way my clothes fit and the way my hair feels. All I do is promote this program to anyone who will listen to me."

She adds, "I have had so many of my friends try it. They have lost weight and are now sticking to the program."

The best thing about the diet, she says, is how easy it is to follow. "I love it!" she says. "I can't say enough good things about this program."

CAN I GET TOO MUCH LEAD FROM BONE BROTH?

Years ago, a scary study purported to find high levels of lead in homemade chicken bone broth.[5] However, big questions were raised about the accuracy of the study, and follow-up studies came to very reassuring conclusions. For example, the National Food Laboratory tested and retested bone broth from grass-fed beef and pastured cows and found no lead in either one.[6] And a study in *Food Additives and Contaminants* found only very small traces of lead in beef bone broth and determined that these primarily came from the tap water

BANISH THE BLOAT!

The foods on the 10-Day Belly Slimdown and Slim Belly Forever Plan will help you gain control over that annoying and unattractive belly bloat. And here's a bonus list of foods to avoid, even after your diet—if you have a special day coming up and you don't want belly bloat to ruin it.

TEN BELLY BLOATERS TO AVOID

Beans

Bubbly alcohol drinks (beer, champagne) and mixers (seltzer, sparkling water)

Dairy foods

Gluten-containing grains

High-salt foods

Artificial sweeteners

Soft drinks

Sugar/high-fructose corn syrup

Sugar-loaded fruits (apples, pears)

Very-high-fiber veggies (good for you, but go easy on red-letter days!)

TEN AWESOME BLOAT-BUSTERS

Replace these with foods that help keep bloat at bay.

Asparagus

Avocado

Bone broth

Cayenne pepper

Celery

Cucumbers

Fermented foods (sauerkraut, kimchi)

Ginger

Green tea

Lemon

used for the broth.[7] (That's why I recommend using filtered water.) So there's no reason to worry.

AFTER I'VE LOST ALL THE WEIGHT I WANT TO LOSE, SHOULD I GO BACK TO A NORMAL EATING WINDOW?

Based on the results I see in my practice, I'd encourage you to keep your eating window as short as you comfortably can. You don't need to keep it as short as you will during the diet, but try eating all your meals within an eight- to twelve-hour window. This will give your body lots of time to burn off fat and "detox" itself.

HEADS UP: WHAT TO EXPECT

Over the last two decades, I've helped thousands of people lose their extra belly fat. As a result, I know all the keys for making a diet succeed. And the biggest key is to *know what to expect*—so that's what this chapter is all about.

First, I'm going to tell you what results you can expect from the diet, based on your body type. These results aren't cast in stone—people often surprise me by losing more pounds and inches than I predict—but they'll give you a good idea of the goals you can shoot for.

Also, because I've guided so many transformations, I have a good feel for what happens at each phase of my diet. So I'm going to tell you what you can anticipate, day by day, on your ten-day adventure. That way, you won't freak out if you feel witchy-and-bitchy on Day 5 or actually gain a pound or two on Day 8. (Don't worry . . . it's all normal!)

And finally, I'm going to introduce you to two culprits that can

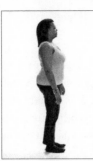
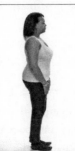

BEFORE   AFTER

RENITA FOSTER

WEIGHT LOST: 6.8 POUNDS | BELLY INCHES LOST: 1.75

Renita says that as a result of the diet, "I have pep in my step."

She adds, "I feel for once I'm doing something good for my body that is sustainable. This isn't so 'faddish' that I am going to tire of it. It just makes so much sense to live this way. I really appreciate what I'm putting into my body now. More important, I'm proud of what I'm not putting into my body."

What would she tell her friends? "PLEASE give it a try. It's sooooo doable. You will feel amazing! Like you've added a few years to your life."

derail even the best diet. The good news is that if you're prepared for them, they'll have zero power over you.

Ready? Here goes.

Factoring in Your Body Type

You know the phrase "Results may vary"? That's definitely true when it comes to dieting. Every person and every body is unique, so two people can follow exactly the same plan and get two very different results.

One factor that plays an especially big role in determining how much weight and how many inches you'll lose on this diet is your body type:

- If you're an "apple," you carry most of your weight around your belly, while your butt, hips, and thighs are slimmer by comparison. On the downside, that visceral fat on your belly is more dangerous than the fat in other areas—but on the upside, it's very metabolically active, and you can burn it off fast. The shortened eating window and the low-carb foods you'll eat on this diet are especially effective for your body type.

- If you're a "pear," you carry more fat on your butt, hips, and thighs than on your belly. That's a good thing when it comes to your health, but it's harder to get this fat to budge than it is to burn belly fat—so you may lose fewer pounds than your apple-shaped diet buddies. Pay extra attention to the Deep Breathing exercise in Chapter 9, which is easy to do when you're dieting and will boost your metabolism so you burn off more weight.

- If you're an "hourglass," you tend to gain or lose weight evenly all over your body. On this diet, you'll lose belly fat and slim down in your arms, butt, thighs, hips, chest, and legs, as well. So expect to keep that hourglass figure . . . only it'll be a slimmer hourglass!

- If you're a "pencil" shape and you're still battling a big belly, there's a good chance you have "cortisol tire" due to stress. In this case, I want you to focus even more intensely than other dieters on the stress-busting tips in Chapter 10. You've got to get control over your stress if you want to shrink that tire.

- If you're an "upside-down pear"—also known as an "inverted triangle"—expect to lose some excess weight on the upper half of your body (bye-bye, arm flab!), as well as on your belly. Lifting weights after you finish your diet will help you trim and tone those arms after you slim them down.

ARE YOUR HORMONES PUTTING POUNDS ON YOU?

One thing that truly can throw a monkey wrench into your weight-loss efforts is a sex hormone imbalance. What's more, these imbalances don't happen only in middle age; in reality, they can start as early as your late twenties or early thirties. This may be the underlying culprit if you're suffering symptoms like these:

- Rapid weight gain
- Loss of interest in sex
- Fatigue
- Brain fog
- Thinning hair
- Breast tenderness
- Mood swings
- Fluid retention
- Insomnia
- Vaginal dryness

Problems with thyroid hormones also can make it tough to lose weight and make you feel miserable all over.

If it turns out that your hormones are wonky, you'll want to tackle the problem before you try to lose your belly fat. Before you start your diet, consider checking your hormones to make sure they are in order. You can order these tests at YourLabWork.com/Dr-Kellyann. If you uncover a problem, find a doctor who is knowledgeable about natural solutions, including bioidentical hormones. These are natural, not synthetic, hormones, and they're safer for your body.

What to Expect on Your Diet, Day by Day

Lots of my patients think I'm psychic. That's because when they're dieting, I say such things as, "Tomorrow you're going to feel bloated," or, "In a day or two, you're going to feel like hitting someone"—and my predictions almost always come true.

However, I don't have any psychic powers; I've simply guided people on this path so many times that I know every twist, turn, and bump in it. And I want you to know about each one, as well, so you won't be caught by surprise!

Here's a quick peek at what you can expect day by day if you follow the typical pattern. And you don't need to take my word for it; these are real comments from the people in my test panel group, along with the advice I gave them.

DAY 1: "I was mentally preparing myself with self-pep-talks—'You got this' kind of stuff—plus imagining what it would be like to be down ten pounds in just over a week. I was nervous about being hungry, and I was little apprehensive about having to make all the shakes and broths with greens."

Dr. Kellyann's advice: It's typical to cycle between being excited and being nervous on Day 1—just like you do at the start of any adventure! This is a good time to talk with supportive peeps who'll keep you inspired.

DAY 2: "Early on, I was thinking, 'This isn't too bad.' I think I was feeling really positive. Later in the day it felt rough, but I just went to bed."

Dr. Kellyann's advice: Around the end of Day 2, the excitement starts to wear off, and that ten-day mark starts to seem pretty far away. Hang in there, and reread your notes about why you're undertaking this challenge. Also, make sure you're drinking plenty of broth and including those healthy fats in your meals.

DAYS 3 AND 4: "These two days were the worst, and I really wanted to punch you (no offense). I felt like I was just white-knuckling

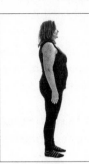

BEFORE   AFTER

DOREEN MARTIN

WEIGHT LOST: 8.2 POUNDS | BELLY INCHES LOST: 1.25

Doreen says, "Bone broth was new to me. I like how easy the diet was to follow." She feels terrific about jump-starting her weight loss and plans to lose more on my 21-Day Bone Broth Diet.

it. Someone in the group said they had a headache on Days 3 and 4."

Dr. Kellyann's advice: This is the "carb flu" I'm going to talk about later in this chapter. Remember: It's temporary, and it's your signal that your body is switching from burning sugar to burning fat. This is the biggest key to blasting your belly fat, so it's a great sign! Also, remember that if you're in your eating window, you can have a few bites of avocado, a handful of unsweetened coconut chips, or some rinsed olives to perk you up.

DAY 5: "One person in our group wrote that they felt amazing on this day. And I commented, 'I'm feeling amazing, too! And I've lost several pounds already, and my body feels less puffy.'"

Dr. Kellyann's advice: You may hit this happy stage a little sooner or later in your own diet—but when you do, you're going to feel like the Energizer bunny. Many of my patients also tell me that they feel "friskier," so you might plan on a little romance!

DAY 6: "Felt some hunger on this day, but I think I felt like I was approaching the top of the hill on a long hike. Told myself I had completed more days than I had left."

Dr. Kellyann's advice: This is a big milestone. Treat yourself to something special—a book, some bubble bath, or a new pair of shoes—to celebrate being more than halfway done.

DAY 7: "Someone in our group said, 'I feel bloated and have a slight headache.' Another person said, 'My sugar cravings subsided, and I don't feel hungry at all.'"

Dr. Kellyann's advice: Ah, the bloat. This may kick in around Day 7 or 8, because you're changing your body's internal ecosystem—firing up good microbes, kicking out bad ones, and adjusting to a diet that's higher in fiber. As a result, you may temporarily experience bloating, diarrhea, or constipation. This "internal housekeeping" stage will pass quickly, so don't kill me if your waistline actually feels a little bigger for a day or two.

DAYS 8 AND 9: "At this point I was in the home stretch, not feeling too hungry, no real cravings, so it felt like that last sprint to the finish where you find fresh drive to get there."

Dr. Kellyann's advice: Right now, you're probably experiencing three emotions: joy that your belly is smaller, excitement that you're nearing the finish line, and a little bit of fear about whether you'll keep that belly fat off. But you don't need to be scared. You know me now . . . I've got you covered! Once you finish your diet, I'll introduce you to my Slim Belly Forever plan, which will keep those pounds off for good without forcing you to starve or give up your favorite foods. From this point on, food won't control you. You now understand not only how different foods *taste,* but how they make you *feel,* and this is life-changing. No more aimless eating. Eating now will be a choice, not a cheat.

DAY 10: "By the last day, I had really found my groove, and hunger was gone . . . like ALL hunger."

Dr. Kellyann's advice: Congratulations—you did it! You're a 10-Day

Belly Slimdown graduate, and you're slim, beautiful, and radiant. Send me some selfies—I can't wait to see how fabulous you look!

With this sneak preview of your ten days, you can tackle your diet confidently. And now, are you ready to meet the two "diet foes" that will try to derail you? Here's a look at each one.

Foe #1: The Sugar Demon

We're genetically wired to love sugar; in fact, it's actually addictive. (Now you know why it's so hard to turn down that candy bar!)

This used to be a good thing, because for our early ancestors, sugar was scarce and came in the healthy forms of berries and honey. So back then, eating sugar was pro-survival. Now, however, sugar is everywhere, and it's packaged in all kinds of junk food that makes us sick.

Worse yet, a few decades ago, scientists figured out a way to make sugar from corn, creating what's called high-fructose corn syrup. Our politicians loved the idea, because 50% of our sugar came from countries selling us sugarcane; now we could make more sugar ourselves. Farmers liked the idea, as well, because getting incentives to grow more corn sounded good. And food manufacturers loved high-fructose corn syrup because it was a cheaper alternative to cane sugar. It was also such a good preservative that they began adding it to foods that hadn't had sugar in them before.

And what did we consumers think? We loved it! After all, it was even sweeter than regular sugar, so we were hooked.

As a result, we're now consuming more sugar than ever. Researchers analyzing data from the Centers for Disease Control estimate that by the year 2050, 95% of the U.S. population will be obese or overweight, mostly due to excessive sugar intake.[1]

What's the answer? Well, you won't like this—but the best solution is to go cold turkey and cut sugar completely out of your diet. At first, you might think that life without sugar isn't worth living. But believe it or not, when you cut sugar out of your diet, you'll eventually stop craving it.

Luckily, right now, I'm not asking you to make a lifelong commitment. I'm just asking you for ten days. (You can do that, right?) What's more, I have some powerful tips that will help you face down that sugar demon. Here they are:

- The average craving lasts only three minutes, so distract yourself by playing a game on your phone, taking a walk, or calling a friend.

- Protein and fat help quell cravings, so drink a cup of bone broth, or—if you're in your eating window—eat a few rinsed olives, a tiny bit of avocado, or some unsweetened coconut chips.

- Try a technique called *urge surfing*. A psychologist named G. Alan Marlatt came up with this years ago, and it's awesome. (It's a lot like mindful meditation, which I talk about on page 196.)

    Here's how it works: When a craving strikes, instead of fighting it, *acknowledge* it in a nonjudgmental way. First, identify where you're feeling the craving most strongly. Is it in your belly, your mouth, or elsewhere? Pay attention to that area, and notice the sensations you're experiencing, such as warmth or tingling.

    Now, pay attention to your breathing for a minute or two, and then shift your attention back to the area where you experienced the craving. Alternate focusing on your breathing and on the area in which you feel the craving. As the craving increases and decreases, picture it as a wave you're riding. Realize that eventually you'll reach the shore, and that craving will be gone.

    The more you practice this technique, the easier it will get for you to resist cravings. It's especially effective if you combine it with regular sessions of mindful meditation.

- When you experience a particularly powerful craving, immediately stop what you're doing and think of a way to commit a random act of kindness—whether it's e-mailing your mom to say hi, ordering a bouquet of flowers for a friend who's feeling low, or calling your sweetie and saying "I love you." The time it takes to plan your act of kindness, along with the warm-and-fuzzy feeling you get from performing it, will help banish your craving.

Above all, keep your mind on how happy you'll be at the end of ten days. Think about the sexy clothes you'll be able to wear—and about the fun of showing off your new flat belly on the beach, at a party, or (ahem) in bed. That's better than a candy bar or a cookie any day, right?

Foe #2: The "Carb Flu"

On this diet, you're going to flip your fat-burning switch from "off" to "on." That's because when you cut out the carbs, your cells will start burning fat instead of sugar for fuel. As a result, you'll become an awesome *fat-burning machine*.

Flipping this switch is the key to nuking your belly fat. It's the solution you've been seeking ever since you first looked at your belly in a dressing-room mirror and said, "Oh, crap."

However . . .

Flipping your switch to fat-burning mode can result in temporary symptoms I call "carb flu." It's not fun, but the good news is that it goes away fast—and if you're ready for it, it won't kill your diet.

Here's the deal. Right now, if you're eating a diet that's high in carbs, your cells are lazy. You're constantly bathing them in sugar, so they don't need to work hard to get the fuel they need.

Burning fat takes more work, and at first your cells will be ticked off about this. As a result, for three to seven days, you may feel tired, cranky, wired, and weird. This isn't fun, but it's actually a great sign—because it tells you that you're switching over to rapid fat-burning mode.

Here's a look at some of the symptoms you may experience when the "carb flu" sets in.

HOW SUGAR IS MAKING YOU LOOK
OLD . . . AND WHY IT MIGHT KILL YOU

Want more reasons to give up your sugar fix? I'm happy to oblige!

- Sugar ages your skin big-time. When you eat sugar, it reacts with amino acids to form compounds called *advanced glycation end products*, or AGEs. These prematurely age your skin, leading to age spots, wrinkles, sags, and bags. Seriously—ick.

    In one interesting study, researchers asked participants to look at photos of a group of people of similar ages who had varying levels of blood glucose. The viewers rated diabetics as looking older than nondiabetics—and among nondiabetics, the researchers say, "Higher glucose levels were correlated with a higher perceived age."[2]

    So here's another trick to try when you have a craving: Think of that cookie or candy bar as a wrinkle waiting to happen, or picture people looking at a photo of you and saying, "Wow . . . *she* hasn't aged well." I bet that sweet treat will instantly look a lot less appealing.

- Sugar ups your risk for cancer. A 2016 study of mice by researchers at the MD Anderson Cancer Center found that diets high in sugar can markedly increase the risk for breast cancer development and metastasis.[3]

- Sugar hurts your heart and blood vessels. Researchers report that people who eat the most sugar are nearly *three times* more likely to die from cardiovascular disease than those eating the least.[4] Even people in the middle range have a one-third higher risk compared to the sugar shunners. This is true even when weight and exercise are factored in.

- Sugar messes with your telomeres. Telomeres are the protective end caps on your DNA. (Think of them as a little like the caps, or aglets, that keep your shoelaces from unraveling.) Researchers at UC San Francisco found that the telomeres in white blood cells of people who drink lots of sugary soda are shorter. The result, the researchers explain, is "accelerated cellular aging of tissues."[5]

I could go on—sugar can also mess with your cholesterol, up your risk for rheumatoid arthritis, and give you belly bloat—but I think you get the picture. In many ways, this addictive white powder is as bad for you as cocaine. It's time to get this monkey off your back!

- You may feel tired. It's perfectly normal to run out of steam on "carb flu" days. If you can, keep your schedule light, and maybe even take a nap or go to bed early. A little coffee can help, but don't overdose on it or you'll feel worse.

- You may feel "flu-ish." You might feel tired or foggy-headed or get the sniffles. But it's not really a bug; it's just a temporary system overhaul.

- You may get moody. Your brain isn't happy right now, because it's used to that heavy load of sugar and carbs. This moodiness, by the way, is related to your changing blood sugar levels. As you continue to eat real foods, you'll get your blood sugar under control and feel happy again.

- You may feel "icky." Digestive disturbances, allergies, and even a little acne may appear at this time. Remember that this is your body removing toxins and healing itself. At the end, you'll be rewarded with a smaller belly, clearer skin, glossier hair, and glowing health.

The key to getting through the "carb flu" is to know why it's happening and understand that it's temporary. Once you're past it, your body will burn fat effortlessly, and you'll feel like a million bucks.

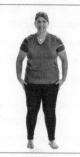
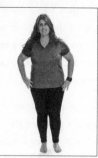

BEFORE   AFTER

MONICA MIRZA

WEIGHT LOST: 8.4 POUNDS | BELLY INCHES LOST: 1.5

Monica says, "I enjoyed all the food and the broth, I never felt hungry, and it was smooth sailing for me. I had no problems." She's happy with her beautiful skin, and she's even more delighted that she slept well during her diet. "I've had horrible problems sleeping through the night," she says, "so this really helped."

In the meantime, you can take steps to make the "carb flu" easier on you. Here are three tips for easing your symptoms:

- If you're hungry during this time, and you're within your eating window, eat a handful of unsweetened coconut chips, a few pieces of avocado, or some olives with the salt rinsed off. (Rinsing olives is a good idea in general, because it reduces your intake of salt, which can bloat you.) This little "hit" of fat can make you feel better fast.

- Journal every day. This will help you spot the signs of "carb flu" and recognize when it's over.

- Diet with a friend if you can. You can give each other moral support when the "carb flu" strikes and remind each other that it'll soon be history.

REMEMBER THESE KEYS TO SUCCESS

KEEP YOUR "EATING WINDOW" SHORT

Condensing your eating into a short window of time will be one of your biggest keys to success, so don't fudge on your timing. If you absolutely need to change a meal-time due to an emergency, get right back on track the next day.

PREP YOUR BROTH, PROTEINS, VEGGIES, BERRIES, AND SHAKES

When you're dashing around in the morning, or you're tired after a busy day, batch prep will make your meal preparation a snap. See Chapter 4 for info on batch cooking before you start your diet.

GET FRIENDS AND FAMILY ON BOARD

Let everyone know ahead of time that you're doing the diet, and ask them to support you. (See Chapter 10 for advice on dealing with people who may try to sabotage you instead.)

AVOID ALCOHOL

I know it's tempting, but even one drink can derail your diet, so stay strong. You can celebrate with a glass of champagne when you're done!

RESIST CHEATS

If the "carb flu" strikes, and you're within your eating window, you can eat a handful of rinsed olives, a few pieces of avocado, or a handful of unsweetened coconut chips. Be careful to avoid any foods that aren't on the plan.

GO EASY ON YOURSELF

If you're used to doing intense workouts, you may want to give yourself a break while you're on your diet. Listen to your body, and rest if you need to. If you're full of energy, try the workouts in Chapter 9. If not, stick to walking or other gentle exercise.

Game On!

At this point, you know what to eat and what not to eat on your diet. You know what to expect on each day of your diet. And you know about the two enemies that will try to sabotage you and how to stop them.

In short, you're ready for action . . . and nothing can stop you. Pick your starting day, do your batch prep (see Chapter 4), and let's *blast that belly fat!*

PART II

BELLY-BLASTING BROTHS, SHAKES, AND MEALS

These easy and delicious recipes will burn the fat off you like *crazy* while they quell your cravings and keep you satisfied from head to toe. With dozens of recipes to choose from, every meal will be a new adventure— and your meal prep will be super easy with my batch-cooking tips, shopping lists, and ten-day meal plan.

4

MAKE IT A CINCH WITH A LITTLE PREP

To kiss your belly fat goodbye, you need to eat the right foods—and you can't get those foods from a fast-food restaurant or a prefab meal in a grocery store freezer.

Instead, you're going to be eating clean, natural foods for the next ten days. And I'll be honest: That's not as effortless as grabbing a burger and fries or tossing a plastic container into the microwave. However, I have a simple solution for you: *batch prep*.

Batch prep is a huge trend these days, because more and more people want to eat right—but who has time to cook every day? The smart way to solve this problem is to do some work ahead of time, buying or cooking lots of the foods you'll need. That way, you'll have a *fully-loaded fridge, freezer, and pantry* waiting for you when it's time to cook or eat.

Note that you have two options:

- A super-easy (ALMOST) NO-COOKING option. With this option, you'll only need to whip up some easy salad dressings and cook a burger one night. Otherwise, you'll buy everything ready-to-go at the store or online. How simple is that?

- A FUN-IN-THE-KITCHEN option. With this option, you'll spend a few hours in the kitchen batch cooking so you'll have meals ready to eat when you want them. (Invite some friends over and make it a batch-cooking party!)

It'll take you a little time to cook or shop for everything you need—but once you're done with this list, *your meals for the entire ten days will be nearly done.* Nice, right?

Option 1: (Almost) No Cooking

With this option, nearly all your prep involves shopping—so you can head straight for your shopping list on page 85.

Two notes before you go shopping:

- You're going to go through a lot of bone broth for this diet plan, so be sure to get plenty of this "liquid gold." Don't skimp on the amount on your shopping list.

- Over the course of your ten-day plan, you'll make a few dressings for your evening SLIM Plate meals. They're delicious and take only three to five minutes to prepare.

Option 2: Fun in the Kitchen

Note: This batch-cooking plan is for one dieter.

Here's how to prepare for the first five days using the meal plan on page 88:

- You're going to need a lot of *bone broth* for this diet plan, so make a double batch of one of the broth recipes before you start. (If you start to run low, it's easy to prepare another batch during your diet days, so keep extra bones on hand.)

- Roast a chicken or buy a rotisserie chicken that does not have sugar or dextrose added (see Roast Chicken with Herbs and Lemon on page 135).

- Make Chicken Vegetable Soup (page 102) and Spicy Mexican Soup (page 112). If you decide not to make these broth loading soups, you can enjoy bone broth with your favorite greens during the broth loading period of the day.

- Make the Asparagus and Tomato Salad (page 144).

- Make the Spicy Coleslaw (page 144).

- Make the No-Bean Chili (page 159) for Days 5 and 7 and freeze it pre-portioned, or prepare it later in the week. You'll only need half the recipe for your food plan, but if you choose, make the full recipe and freeze it pre-portioned for later.

- On Day 4, prepare the Creamy Broccoli Soup (page 104) that you'll enjoy on Days 5 and 7. You can also prepare this ahead and freeze it if it's easier for you.

On Day 4 or 5 you can begin preparing for the next five days:

- Keep that bone broth simmering!

- Make Watercress Soup (page 114) and Creamy Tomato Florentine Soup (page 108). If you decide not to make these broth loading soups, you can enjoy bone broth with your favorite greens during the Broth Loading period of the day.

- Prepare Unstuffed Cabbage (page 166). You'll only need half the recipe for your food plan, but if you choose, make the full recipe and freeze it pre-portioned for later.

- Prepare Lemon Rosemary Chicken with Cauliflower "Rice" (page 158) or wait until Day 8. It's quick and easy to make. You'll only need half the recipe for your food plan, but if you choose, make the full recipe and freeze it pre-portioned for later.

Your Ten-Day Meal Plan

This meal plan uses the foods you've batch cooked or bought. Here's how it works:

- In the SLIM Plate sections of these meal plans, you'll find options for both cooked and no-cook (or almost no-cook) meals.

- In the broth loading phase, you can make a broth loading soup or simply drink broth with leafy greens added.

- In the shake section, you can pick a recipe or simply make your own shake (as long as it follows the rules for shakes).

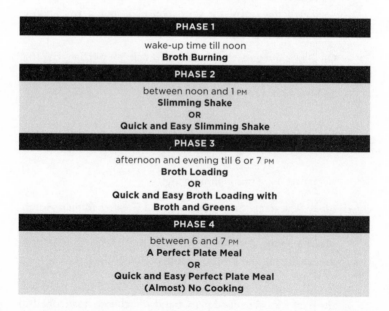

PHASE 1
wake-up time till noon **Broth Burning**

PHASE 2
between noon and 1 PM **Slimming Shake** OR **Quick and Easy Slimming Shake**

PHASE 3
afternoon and evening till 6 or 7 PM **Broth Loading** OR **Quick and Easy Broth Loading with Broth and Greens**

PHASE 4
between 6 and 7 PM **A Perfect Plate Meal** OR **Quick and Easy Perfect Plate Meal (Almost) No Cooking**

NOTE: There's a printable version of this plan on the Resources page on my website, drkellyann.com/gift.

	DAY 1	DAY 2	DAY 3	DAY 4	DAY 5
Broth Burning	Up to 48 ounces bone broth	Up to 48 ounces bone broth	Up to 48 ounces bone broth	Up to 48 ounces bone broth	Up to 48 ounces bone broth
Slimming Shake **OR** **Quick and Easy Slimming Shake**	Chocolate Almond Shake **OR** Create your own shake using meal plan instructions	Chocolate Coconut Shake **OR** Create your own shake using meal plan instructions	Berry Shake **OR** Create your own shake using meal plan instructions	Latte Shake **OR** Create your own shake using meal plan instructions	Chocolate Mint Shake **OR** Create your own shake using meal plan instructions
Broth Loading **OR** **Quick and Easy Broth Loading with Broth and Greens**	Chicken Vegetable Soup **OR** Bone Broth and 2 handfuls of non-starchy veggies using meal plan instructions	Spicy Mexican Soup **OR** Bone Broth and 2 handfuls of non-starchy veggies using meal plan instructions	Chicken Vegetable Soup **OR** Bone Broth and 2 handfuls of non-starchy veggies using meal plan instructions	Spicy Mexican Soup **OR** Bone Broth and 2 handfuls of non-starchy veggies using meal plan instructions	Creamy Broccoli Soup **OR** Bone Broth and 2 handfuls of non-starchy veggies using meal plan instructions
A SLIM Plate Meal **OR** **Quick and Easy SLIM Plate Meal (ALMOST) NO COOKING**	Roast Chicken Asparagus and Tomato Salad ¹/2 grapefruit or handful of berries (optional) **OR** Avocado Tuna Salad ¹/2 grapefruit or handful of berries (optional)	Beef or Turkey Burger Spicy Coleslaw ¹/2 grapefruit or handful of berries (optional) **OR** Turkey Wraps with Green Goddess Dressing ¹/2 grapefruit or handful of berries (optional)	Roast Chicken Asparagus and Tomato Salad ¹/2 grapefruit or handful of berries (optional) **OR** Chicken with Creamy Cilantro Sauce ¹/2 grapefruit or handful of berries (optional)	Roast Chicken Spicy Coleslaw ¹/2 grapefruit or handful of berries (optional) **OR** Cobb Salad ¹/2 grapefruit or handful of berries (optional)	No-Bean Chili ¹/2 grapefruit or handful of berries (optional) **OR** Beef or Turkey Burger with Avocado Cucumber Salad ¹/2 grapefruit or handful of berries (optional)

	DAY 6	DAY 7	DAY 8	DAY 9	DAY 10
Broth Burning	Up to 48 ounces bone broth	Up to 48 ounces bone broth	Up to 48 ounces bone broth	Up to 48 ounces bone broth	Up to 48 ounces bone broth
Slimming Shake	Chocolate Almond Shake	Chocolate Coconut Shake	Berry Shake	Latte Shake	Chocolate Mint Shake
OR	**OR**	**OR**	**OR**	**OR**	**OR**
Quick and Easy Slimming Shake	Create your own shake using meal plan instructions	Create your own shake using meal plan instructions	Create your own shake using meal plan instructions	Create your own shake using meal plan instructions	Create your own shake using meal plan instructions
Broth Loading	Watercress Soup	Creamy Broccoli Soup	Creamy Tomato Florentine Soup	Watercress Soup	Creamy Tomato Florentine Soup
OR	**OR**	**OR**	**OR**	**OR**	**OR**
Quick and Easy Broth Loading with Broth and Greens	Bone Broth and 2 handfuls of non-starchy veggies using meal plan instructions	Bone Broth and 2 handfuls of non-starchy veggies using meal plan instructions	Bone Broth and 2 handfuls of non-starchy veggies using meal plan instructions	Bone Broth and 2 handfuls of non-starchy veggies using meal plan instructions	Bone Broth and 2 handfuls of non-starchy veggies using meal plan instructions
A SLIM Plate Meal	Unstuffed Cabbage 1/2 grapefruit or handful of berries (optional)	No-Bean Chili 1/2 grapefruit or handful of berries (optional)	Lemon Rosemary Chicken with Cauliflower Rice 1/2 grapefruit or handful of berries (optional)	Unstuffed Cabbage 1/2 grapefruit or handful of berries (optional)	Lemon Rosemary Chicken with Cauliflower "Rice" 1/2 grapefruit or handful of berries (optional)
OR	**OR**	**OR**	**OR**	**OR**	**OR**
Quick and Easy SLIM Plate Meal (ALMOST) NO COOKING	Rotisserie Chicken with Avocado Cucumber Salad 1/2 grapefruit or handful of berries (optional)	Chicken Caesar Salad 1/2 grapefruit or handful of berries (optional)	Chipotle Chicken Wraps 1/2 grapefruit or handful of berries (optional)	Butter Lettuce with Avocado Egg Salad 1/2 grapefruit or handful of berries (optional)	Turkey Wraps with Green Goddess Dressing 1/2 grapefruit or handful of berries (optional)

Your Shopping Lists

To make sure you have all the ingredients you'll need for this meal plan, here are two shopping lists—one for the (Almost) No-Cooking option and one for the Fun in the Kitchen option—that will set you up for the entire ten days. Each list is divided into two sections: one section for your first shopping trip, and one section for restocking before your second five days. There are printable versions of these on the Resources page on my website, drkellyann.com/gift, that you can take to the store.

SHOPPING FOR THE (ALMOST) NO-COOKING OPTION

Because this is a ten-day plan, you can shop for all the staples prior to starting and pick up additional produce and meats sometime between Days 4 and 6. You probably have many of the items in your pantry already.

PART 1: ITEMS TO BUY ON YOUR FIRST SHOPPING TRIP (STOCKING UP FOR DAYS 1 THROUGH 5)

BROTH AND SHAKES

AT LEAST FOUR GALLONS OF BROTH TO START. See tips for buying bone broth on page 41.

PROTEIN POWDERS (10 servings total for the entire meal plan):

DR. KELLYANN'S CHOCOLATE BONE BROTH PROTEIN POWDER or ANOTHER HIGH-QUALITY CHOCOLATE BEEF PROTEIN (15 to 25 grams protein/serving; see tips for selecting a high-quality product on page 42)

and/or

DR. KELLYANN'S VANILLA BONE BROTH PROTEIN POWDER or ANOTHER HIGH-QUALITY VANILLA BEEF PROTEIN (15 to 25 grams protein/serving; see tips for selecting a high-quality product on page 42)

FATS

There are lots of fat options you can enjoy, and the choice is yours. Those with asterisks are required for the meal plan. You can also buy any of the others listed here for variety.

CANNED FULL-FAT COCONUT MILK

COCONUT OIL

MCT OIL

OLIVE OIL*

AVOCADO OIL*

WALNUT OIL

CHIA SEEDS

GROUND FLAXSEED

HEMP SEEDS

AVOCADOS (see the produce list)

UNSWEETENED ALMOND BUTTER

PASTURE-RAISED BUTTER

GHEE (page 147)

AVOCADO OIL MAYONNAISE*

HERBS, SEASONINGS, AND OTHER PANTRY ITEMS

MONK FRUIT SWEETENER OR STEVIA (optional)

BALSAMIC VINEGAR

DIJON MUSTARD

CUMIN

DILL

CAYENNE PEPPER

CRUSHED RED PEPPER (optional)

CAPERS (optional)

CELTIC OR PINK HIMALAYAN SALT

BLACK PEPPER

COCONUT AMINOS

TUNA IN WATER (one 5-ounce can)

ANCHOVY PASTE (1 small tube)

CHIPOTLE IN ADOBO SAUCE (1 small can)

BEVERAGES

UNSWEETENED ALMOND MILK (carrageenan-free) OR COCONUT MILK (not canned; 1/2 gallon)

SPARKLING WATER

COFFEE AND/OR MY COLLAGEN COFFEE

TEA—BLACK, GREEN, WHITE, OR HERBAL

PRODUCE

BLUEBERRIES

GRAPEFRUIT

LEAFY GREENS (Since you can have up to 6 cups of broth, you can have up to 12 handfuls of greens with it. Ultimately you can have up to 14 cups of greens per day.)

AVOCADOS (3 or 4)

CELERY (1 stalk)

RED ONION (1)

ONIONS (2)

RADISHES (1 bunch)

LEMONS (3)

LARGE-LEAF LETTUCE SUCH AS BIBB OR ROMAINE (1 head)

LETTUCE OF YOUR CHOICE FOR 2 SALADS (1 to 2 heads/bunches)

TOMATOES (3)

CUCUMBERS (4)

CILANTRO (2 bunches)

LIMES (2)

GARLIC (2 heads)

TARRAGON (1 bunch)

CHIVES (1 bunch)

PARSLEY (1 bunch)

MEAT AND EGGS

1 ROTISSERIE CHICKEN (*Note:* You probably won't eat the entire chicken— you can freeze the rest for the next week.)

4 OUNCES SLICED DELI TURKEY BREAST, SUGAR-, NITRITE-, AND NITRATE-FREE

1 HARD-BOILED EGG

6 OUNCES GROUND BEEF, SIRLOIN, OR TURKEY FOR A BURGER

PART 2: ITEMS TO BUY ON YOUR SECOND SHOPPING TRIP (STOCKING UP FOR DAYS 6 THROUGH 10)

BEVERAGES

UNSWEETENED ALMOND MILK (carrageenan-free) OR COCONUT MILK (not canned; 1/2 gallon)

PRODUCE

Before shopping for Days 6 through 10, check for any produce left from Days 1 through 5.

BLUEBERRIES

GRAPEFRUIT

LEAFY GREENS

ROMAINE LETTUCE (2 heads)

LARGE BEEFSTEAK TOMATO (1 large or 2 or 3 smaller tomatoes)

BASIL (1 bunch)

AVOCADO (1)

BUTTER OR BIBB LETTUCE (1 head)

CUCUMBER (1)

LIME (1)

LEMON (1)

MEAT AND EGGS

1 ROTISSERIE CHICKEN

1 TO 3 HARD-BOILED EGGS

4 OUNCES SLICED DELI TURKEY BREAST, SUGAR-, NITRITE-, AND NITRATE-FREE

SHOPPING FOR THE FUN-IN-THE-KITCHEN OPTION

Because this is a 10-day plan, you can shop for all the staples prior to starting and pick up additional produce and meats sometime between days 4 and 6. You probably have many of the spices and dry goods in your pantry already.

PART 1: ITEMS TO BUY ON YOUR FIRST SHOPPING TRIP (STOCKING UP FOR DAYS 1 THROUGH 5)

BONE BROTH INGREDIENTS

Bone broth is a cornerstone of your meal plan, so don't skimp on this! If you make a double recipe of Chicken Bone Broth (page 96) for Days 1 through 5 and again for Days 6 through 10, you'll have about 2 gallons of broth for each five-day period. You may want more broth, since you can have up to 12 cups per day.

After the first two days on the plan, you'll have a sense of how often you'll need to make bone broth. The shopping list below has ingredients to make up to 4 gallons of broth. You also have the option of buying pre-prepared bone broth.

PROTEIN POWDERS/COFFEE POWDERS

10 SERVINGS TOTAL FOR THE ENTIRE MEAL PLAN:

DR. KELLYANN'S CHOCOLATE BONE BROTH PROTEIN POWDER or ANOTHER HIGH-QUALITY CHOCOLATE BEEF PROTEIN (15 to 25 grams protein/serving)—8 servings for the entire meal plan (see tips for selecting a high-quality product on page 42)

DR. KELLYANN'S VANILLA BONE BROTH PROTEIN POWDER or ANOTHER HIGH-QUALITY VANILLA BEEF PROTEIN (15 to 25 grams protein/serving)—2 servings for the entire meal plan (see tips for selecting a high-quality product on page 42)

COLLAGEN COFFEE™ OR ESPRESSO POWDER (1 packet collagen coffee or 1 tablespoon espresso)

FATS

There are lots of fat options you can enjoy, and the choice is yours. Those with asterisks are required for the meal plan. You can also buy any of the others listed here for variety.

CANNED FULL-FAT COCONUT MILK (four 14-ounce cans)*

COCONUT OIL*

MCT OIL

OLIVE OIL*

AVOCADO OIL*

WALNUT OIL

CHIA SEEDS

GROUND FLAXSEED

HEMP SEEDS

AVOCADOS (see the produce list)

UNSWEETENED ALMOND BUTTER*

PASTURE-RAISED BUTTER

GHEE* (you can also make ghee from butter; see page 147)

AVOCADO OIL MAYONNAISE* (you can also make it; see page 117)

HERBS, SEASONINGS, AND OTHER PANTRY ITEMS

MONK FRUIT SWEETENER OR STEVIA (optional)

UNSEASONED RICE VINEGAR

APPLE CIDER VINEGAR

RED WINE VINEGAR

DIJON MUSTARD

PURE VANILLA EXTRACT

PURE MINT EXTRACT

BAY LEAVES

NUTMEG

THYME

CUMIN

CHILI POWDER

OREGANO

CAYENNE PEPPER

GARLIC POWDER

HUNGARIAN PAPRIKA

ITALIAN SEASONING

CRUSHED RED PEPPER

COCONUT AMINOS

ARROWROOT (optional, for thickening sauces)

CANNED DICED TOMATOES (three 28-ounce cans)

BEVERAGES

UNSWEETENED ALMOND MILK (carrageenan-free) OR COCONUT MILK (not canned; 1/2 gallon)

SPARKLING WATER

COFFEE AND/OR MY COLLAGEN COFFEE

TEA—BLACK, GREEN, WHITE, OR HERBAL

PRODUCE

BLUEBERRIES (1 pint fresh or frozen for Berry Shake; *Note:* If you buy frozen or freeze half the pint, you'll have enough for the Berry Shake on Day 8. *Optional:* Get 2 pints if you plan on having blueberries after your SLIM Plate meal.)

SPINACH (2 large boxes of fresh baby spinach; *Note:* You can select from any of the greens listed in the approved foods list; however, spinach adds little to your shake, so 1 large box for shakes is included here.)

GARLIC (2 or 3 heads)

YELLOW ONIONS (5)

RED ONION (1)

BROCCOLI (2 crowns/heads)

CELERY (1 stalk)

GREEN BEANS (about $1/2$ pound)

YELLOW SQUASH (2 small)

RED BELL PEPPERS (2)

CABBAGE (1 small head)

CILANTRO (1 bunch)

THYME (1 bunch)

ROSEMARY (1 bunch; you will use it again on Days 6 through 10; it will stay fresh in the refrigerator.)

PARSLEY (1 bunch; you will use it again on Days 6 through 10; it will stay fresh in the refrigerator.)

FRESH GINGER (1 small knob)

BASIL (1 bunch)

LIME (1)

LEMONS (3)

JALAPEÑO PEPPERS (2)

CARROTS (1 pound; for Bone Broth for all 10 days)

GRAPEFRUIT (3; *Optional:* If you plan on having $1/2$ grapefruit after your SLIM Plate meal.)

ASPARAGUS (1 bunch)

TOMATOES (2)

SCALLIONS (1 bunch)

NAPA OR SAVOY CABBAGE (1 small to medium head, to yield about 4 cups)

YOUR FAVORITE LETTUCE (1 head or 5-ounce bag/plastic box)

CUCUMBER (1)

AVOCADO (1)

ZUCCHINI (4 small)

MEATS

6 POUNDS RAW OR COOKED CHICKEN BONES/CARCASSES (for bone broth)

4 POUNDS CHICKEN THIGHS, LEGS, AND/OR WINGS (for bone broth)

12 TO 16 CHICKEN FEET, OPTIONAL, BUT WILL ADD A GREAT DEAL OF COLLAGEN TO YOUR BROTH (for bone broth)

WHOLE CHICKEN (3 to 4 pounds or 1 rotisserie chicken for Days 1, 3, and 4)

6 OUNCES GROUND BEEF OR TURKEY FOR A BURGER ON DAY 2

$1^1/4$ POUNDS GROUND BEEF OR SIRLOIN FOR NO-BEAN CHILI ON DAYS 5 AND 7

PART 2: ITEMS TO BUY ON YOUR SECOND SHOPPING TRIP (STOCKING UP FOR DAYS 6 THROUGH 10)

BEVERAGES

UNSWEETENED ALMOND MILK (carrageenan-free) OR COCONUT MILK (not canned; 1/2 gallon)

PRODUCE

Before shopping for Days 6 through 10, check for any produce left from Days 1 through 5.

BLUEBERRIES (*Optional:* Get 2 pints if you plan on having blueberries after your SLIM Plate meal.)

SPINACH (1 large plastic box or bag baby spinach and 1 small box or bag; *Note:* You can select from any of the greens listed in the approved foods list; however, spinach adds little to no flavor to your shake, so 1 large box for shakes is included here.)

WATERCRESS (2 or more 14-ounce or larger bunches)

BASIL (1 bunch)

BUTTER LETTUCE (1 head)

AVOCADO (1)

TOMATO (1)

CABBAGE (1 large head or about 8 cups pre-cut cabbage)

ONIONS (3)

CAULIFLOWER (1 head or 1 bag cauliflower "rice")

GRAPEFRUIT (2 or 3; *Optional:* If you plan on having 1/2 grapefruit after your SLIM Plate meal.)

MEAT

6 POUNDS RAW OR COOKED CHICKEN BONES/CARCASSES (for bone broth)

4 POUNDS CHICKEN THIGHS, LEGS, AND/OR WINGS (for bone broth)

12 TO 16 CHICKEN FEET, OPTIONAL, BUT WILL ADD A GREAT DEAL OF COLLAGEN TO YOUR BROTH (for bone broth)

6 BONELESS, SKINLESS CHICKEN THIGHS FOR LEMON ROSEMARY CHICKEN ON DAYS 8 AND 10

1 1/4 POUNDS GROUND BEEF OR SIRLOIN FOR UNSTUFFED CABBAGE (page 166) ON DAYS 6 AND 9

So there you go: Bookmark the meal plan so you can find it easily, take a quick trip to the store to load up on everything you'll need, and do a little batch prep. Then pat yourself on the back, because you've set yourself up for success!

BUST IT OUT WITH BONE BROTH

Now that you know all about luscious, satisfying bone broth—my fat-blasting "liquid gold"—I know you're eager to make your first batch. And I can't wait for you to try it!

In this chapter, you'll find a wealth of recipes for basic broths and spice-packed variations to enjoy during your "broth burning" phase, as well as veggie-rich broths for your "broth loading" phase. Take your pick, because every single recipe is loaded with fat-burning power.

And before you start, I want to reassure you about something: *You really can't do this wrong.*

After I wrote *Dr. Kellyann's Bone Broth Diet,* I got thousands of e-mails from dieters who worried they'd cooked their broth too long or not long enough. I also got e-mails from dieters who were afraid they'd picked the wrong bones or that their broth wasn't jiggly enough. (Bone broth normally jiggles when you chill it because of the gelatin in it.)

Seriously, people were freaking out.

Well, I'm going to tell you exactly what I told them: Relax!

I'm going to give you some tips for making the best broth, but you don't need to obsess over this. If you can throw half a dozen ingredients into a sturdy stockpot and turn on a stove burner, you're good to go. Trust me: It's not rocket science.

I mean, think about it. The earliest humans made bone broth over a fire while wearing animal skins. And we're talking about people who'd barely *discovered* fire. Clearly, it's not that hard.

That said, there are some tricks for getting the most nutrition and "jiggle" from your broth. Here they are:

- Buy bones with lots of cartilage. Chicken drumsticks or whole carcasses are great; so are beef knuckle, joint, and marrow bones. If you're not sure which bones are best, simply ask your butcher. He or she can also special-order bones for you.

- Experiment to find the right amount of time to cook your broth. If it doesn't turn out jiggly when chilled, try reducing or increasing your cooking time the next time. (If you cook broth too long, it can break down the collagen building blocks to the point that they lose their "jiggle." Conversely, if you don't cook it long enough, you won't pull enough gelatin out of the bones to get the wobble you want.)

- Use just enough water to cover the bones.

- Keep your broth at a low simmer.

These tips should help you produce a perfect pot of jiggly bone broth. But even if yours doesn't turn out perfect, it's fine! Jiggle or no jiggle, as long as you've cooked it for the minimum amount of time, it'll be loaded with gelatin and other fat-melting nutrients.

In short, don't be the least bit intimidated by the idea of making bone broth. It's incredibly easy to make, and yours will be fabulous. So relax . . . and get cooking!

A Few Additional Tips

The biggest key to making great bone broth is to become BFFs with your butcher, so don't be shy about getting to know the butchers at your favorite stores.

In addition to making friends with your local butchers, you can find great bones by searching online for ranchers who sell them. Type in *grass fed bones,* and you're likely to find some great resources nearby.

If you can afford it, use bones from pastured animals. If not, don't sweat it. Just remove the skin from poultry or the fat from meat, because that's where toxins accumulate.

To add more flavor to your beef broth, get some meaty bones such as oxtails, shanks, and short ribs. And to make any broth more flavorful, you can add chicken feet. (If that grosses you out, relax . . . you don't need to do it.)

If you're on a tight budget, here's a good trick: Reuse beef or poultry bones. You can get at least two batches of broth out of them.

For fish-bone broth, buy high-quality, wild-caught fish. Avoid oily fish such as salmon and mackerel, which can develop off flavors if you cook them for a long time. Instead, pick nonoily fish such as sole, snapper, halibut, turbot, tilapia, cod, or rockfish. Often, fish markets clean their own fish and throw away the bones, so ask if they'd be willing to save them for you.

Recipes for Your "Broth Burning" and "Broth Loading" Phases

In the first section here, you'll find basic broths for your morning phase. You'll also use these broths as the base for your afternoon recipes.

BEEF BONE BROTH

PREP TIME: **15 MIN.** | COOK TIME: **3 TO 12 HRS. DEPENDING ON COOKING MODE** |
YIELD: **ABOUT 1 GALLON OF BROTH**

3 pounds or more beef bones
(see Note)

2 pounds or more meaty bones
such as oxtail, short ribs, etc.

1/4 cup apple cider vinegar

2 ripe tomatoes, cut into wedges

2 to 4 carrots, roughly chopped

3 or 4 celery ribs, including
leaves, roughly chopped

1 medium onion, cut into large
wedges

1 or 2 garlic cloves

2 bay leaves

2 teaspoons Celtic or pink
Himalayan salt

1 teaspoon whole black
peppercorns

Filtered water

FAT-BURNING SPICES (ADD FOR MORE FAT-BURNING POWER)

1 tablespoon instant espresso
powder

1 (1-inch) knob fresh ginger, sliced

Handful of fresh parsley or
cilantro

Ground turmeric (1 teaspoon or
more per gallon)

Cayenne pepper (1/8 teaspoon or
more per gallon)

Ground cumin (1 teaspoon or
more per gallon)

Place all the bones and meat in a large stockpot, slow cooker, pressure cooker, or Instant Pot. Add the vinegar, vegetables, bay leaves, salt, and peppercorns. Add any additional fat-burning spices. Add enough filtered water to cover everything by 1 inch.

If using a stockpot, bring the liquid to a simmer over medium heat, then reduce the heat to low. Cover and let simmer for at least 12 hours, adding filtered water as needed so the bones are always covered.

In a slow cooker, cover and cook on low for at least 12 hours or up to 24 hours, adding filtered water only if needed so the bones are always covered.

In a pressure cooker or Instant Pot, using your cooker's instructions, bring to full pressure. Reduce the heat to low, maintaining full pressure, and cook for 3 hours. Allow the pressure to naturally release.

When the broth is done, strain it through a fine-mesh strainer. Discard the bones and vegetables, and reserve the meat for another use. (Or you can refrigerate or freeze the bones and reuse them to make another batch of broth.)

Set the broth aside to cool, then cover and refrigerate. When chilled, the broth should be very gelatinous. The broth will keep in the refrigerator for up to 5 days or in the freezer for 3 months or more.

NOTE: Joint, neck, and knuckle bones are best because they have the highest amount of collagen. Marrow bones are also excellent.

CHICKEN BONE BROTH

PREP TIME: **15 MIN.** | COOK TIME: **2 TO 8 HRS. DEPENDING ON COOKING MODE** | YIELD: **ABOUT 1 GALLON OF BROTH**

3 pounds or more raw or cooked chicken bones/carcasses

2 pounds or more chicken thighs, legs, and/or wings

6 to 8 chicken feet (optional, but will add a great deal of collagen to your broth)

1/4 cup apple cider vinegar

2 to 4 carrots, roughly chopped

3 or 4 celery ribs, including leaves, roughly chopped

1 medium onion, cut into large chunks

1 or 2 garlic cloves

1 bay leaf

2 teaspoons Celtic or pink Himalayan salt

1 teaspoon whole black peppercorns

Filtered water

FAT-BURNING SPICES (ADD FOR MORE FAT-BURNING POWER)

1 (1-inch) knob fresh ginger, sliced

Handful of fresh parsley or cilantro

Ground turmeric (1 teaspoon or more per gallon)

Cayenne pepper (1/8 teaspoon or more per gallon)

Ground cumin (1 teaspoon or more per gallon)

Place all the bones and meat in a large stockpot, slow cooker, pressure cooker, or Instant Pot. Add the chicken feet (if using), vinegar, vegetables, bay leaf, salt, and peppercorns. Add any additional fat-burning spices. Add enough filtered water to cover everything by 1 inch.

If using a stockpot, bring the liquid to a simmer over medium heat, then reduce the heat to low. Cover and let simmer for at least 4 hours or up to 8 hours, adding filtered water as needed so the bones are always covered.

In a slow cooker, cover and cook on low for 8 hours, adding filtered water only if needed so the bones are always covered.

TWO EASY ALTERNATIVES TO THE STOCKPOT

Now that I've talked about how simple it is to make basic bone broth on the stovetop, I want to share two ways to make this project fit easily into your busy schedule.

First, you can make your broth in a slow cooker. The water won't evaporate as it does in a stockpot, so you won't need to tend the broth as much.

Second, if you need broth fast, you can make it in a pressure cooker. Here's how to do it.

- Put all the ingredients in a pressure cooker and add enough filtered water to cover everything by 1 inch. Lock the lid in place.

- Raise the heat to high until the pressure cooker reaches full pressure (10 to 15 minutes). Then set the heat to low and cook for 2 hours if you're using chicken bones and about 3 hours if you're using beef bones. (Fish bones cook so quickly that pressure cooking isn't recommended.)

- When you're done, turn off the heat and let the pressure cooker cool down and release pressure naturally until it's ready to open. When your broth is cool, just strain it, and voilà! You have beautiful broth.

In a pressure cooker or Instant Pot, using your cooker's instructions, bring to full pressure. Reduce the heat to low, maintaining full pressure, and cook for 2 hours. Allow the pressure to naturally release.

When the broth is done, strain it through a fine-mesh strainer. Discard the bones and vegetables, and reserve the meat for another use. (Or you can refrigerate or freeze the bones and reuse them to make another batch of broth.)

Set the broth aside to cool, then cover and refrigerate. When chilled, the broth should be very gelatinous. The broth will keep in the refrigerator for up to 5 days or in the freezer for 3 months or more.

ROTISSERIE CHICKEN BONE BROTH

PREP TIME: **15 MIN.** | COOK TIME: **2 TO 8 HRS. DEPENDING ON COOKING MODE** | YIELD: **ABOUT 1 GALLON OF BROTH**

3 carcasses or more from rotisserie chickens

Drumsticks, thighs, and wings from 1 rotisserie chicken, or 2 pounds or more chicken thighs, legs, and/or wings

6 to 8 chicken feet (optional, but will add a great deal of collagen to your broth)

1/4 cup apple cider vinegar

2 to 4 carrots, roughly chopped

3 or 4 celery ribs, including leaves, roughly chopped

1 medium onion, cut into large chunks

1 or 2 garlic cloves

1 bay leaf

2 teaspoons Celtic or pink Himalayan salt

1 teaspoon whole black peppercorns

Filtered water

FAT-BURNING SPICES (ADD FOR MORE FAT-BURNING POWER)

1 (1-inch) knob fresh ginger, sliced

Handful of fresh parsley or cilantro

Ground turmeric (1 teaspoon or more per gallon)

Cayenne pepper (1/8 teaspoon or more per gallon)

Ground cumin (1 teaspoon or more per gallon)

Place all the bones and meat in a large stockpot, slow cooker, pressure cooker, or Instant Pot. Add the chicken feet (if using), vinegar, vegetables, bay leaf, salt, and peppercorns. Add any additional fat-burning spices. Add enough filtered water to cover everything by 1 inch.

If using a stockpot, bring the water to a simmer over medium heat, then reduce the heat to low. Cover and let simmer for at least 4 hours or up to 8 hours, adding filtered was as needed so the bones are always covered.

In a slow cooker, cover and cook on low for 8 hours, adding filtered water only if needed so the bones are always covered.

In a pressure cooker or Instant Pot, using your cooker's instructions, bring to full pressure. Reduce the heat to low, maintaining full pressure, and cook for 2 hours. Allow the pressure to naturally release.

When the broth is done, strain it through a fine-mesh strainer. Discard the bones and vegetables, and reserve the meat for another use. (Or you can refrigerate or freeze the bones and reuse them to make another batch of broth.)

Set the broth aside to cool, then cover and refrigerate. When chilled, the broth should be very gelatinous. The broth will keep in the refrigerator for up to 5 days or in the freezer for 3 months or more.

GET CREATIVE!

You can spice up any of the bone broth recipes with any of the fat-burning herbs and spices listed on pages 48–50 or any variation of the seasonings to create flavors you enjoy.

For a Chinese-style broth, try a 2-inch knob of fresh ginger (sliced), scallions, lemongrass, cilantro, Chinese five-spice powder, and white pepper.

For a Thai-style broth, try fresh ginger, lemongrass, scallions, makrut lime leaves, galangal, and white pepper.

For a spicy broth with Mexican flavors, add cilantro, cumin, cayenne, cinnamon, coriander, and jalapeños or other chile peppers.

For an Italian-style broth, add tomatoes, Italian seasoning, basil, parsley, marjoram, fennel, aniseed, and oregano.

For a Greek-style broth, try oregano, sage, marjoram, savory, fennel leaves, rosemary, thyme, dill, purslane, and fresh lemon juice.

To add flavors from Provence, try fresh thyme, marjoram, lavender, summer savory, mint, and rosemary.

For Middle Eastern flavors, try sumac, saffron, cilantro, coriander, parsley, mint, turmeric, caraway, aniseed, fenugreek, and allspice.

SEAFOOD BONE BROTH

PREP TIME: **15 MIN.** | COOK TIME: **45 TO 65 MIN.** | YIELD: **ABOUT 1 GALLON OF BROTH**

12 or more shrimp shells and tails

2 pounds or more fish carcasses or heads from large nonoily fish, such as halibut, cod, sole, rockfish, turbot, tilapia, etc.

2 tablespoons ghee (page 147) or pastured butter

2 to 4 carrots, roughly chopped

3 or 4 celery ribs, including leaves, roughly chopped

1 medium onion, cut into large chunks

1 tablespoon pickling spice mix

1 teaspoon whole black peppercorns

Filtered water

FAT-BURNING SPICES (ADD FOR MORE FAT-BURNING POWER)

1 (1-inch) knob fresh ginger, sliced

Handful of fresh Italian parsley or cilantro

Ground turmeric (1 teaspoon or more per gallon)

Cayenne pepper (1/8 teaspoon or more per gallon)

Rinse the shrimp shells and fish carcasses or heads. Cut off the gills.

In a large stockpot, melt the ghee over low heat. Add the carrots, celery, and onion and cook, stirring occasionally, for about 20 minutes, until softened.

Add the fish bones and shrimp shells, pickling spice, peppercorns, and any additional fat-burning spices. Add enough filtered water to cover everything by 1 inch and increase the heat to medium. Bring the water to a bare simmer and reduce the heat to low. Use a shallow spoon to skim the foam off the top of the broth. Cook at a bare simmer, uncovered or with a lid askew, for 25 to 40 minutes. Continue to skim the surface as needed.

When the broth is done, strain it through a fine-mesh strainer. Discard the solids.

Set the broth aside to cool, then cover and refrigerate. When chilled, the broth should be very gelatinous. The broth will keep in the refrigerator for up to 5 days or in the freezer for 3 months or more.

NOTE: Because fish bones are so soft and the cooking process so fast, you should not prepare Seafood Bone Broth in a slow cooker, pressure cooker, or Instant Pot.

TURKEY BONE BROTH

PREP TIME: **15 MIN** | COOK TIME: **2 TO 8 HRS. DEPENDING ON COOKING MODE** |
YIELD: **ABOUT 1 GALLON OF BROTH**

3 pounds or more raw or cooked turkey bones/carcasses

2 pounds or more turkey thighs, legs, and/or wings

6 to 8 chicken feet (optional, but will add a great deal of collagen to your broth)

1/4 cup apple cider vinegar

2 to 4 carrots, roughly chopped

3 or 4 celery ribs, including leaves, roughly chopped

1 medium onion, cut into large chunks

1 or 2 garlic cloves

1 teaspoon dried sage

2 teaspoons Celtic or pink Himalayan salt

1 teaspoon whole black peppercorns

Filtered water

FAT-BURNING SPICES (ADD FOR MORE FAT-BURNING POWER)

1 (1-inch) knob fresh ginger, sliced

Handful of fresh Italian parsley or cilantro

Ground turmeric (1 teaspoon or more per gallon)

Cayenne pepper (1/8 teaspoon or more per gallon)

Ground cumin (1 teaspoon or more per gallon)

Place all the bones and meat in a large stockpot, slow cooker, pressure cooker, or Instant Pot. Add the chicken feet (if using), vinegar, vegetables, sage, salt, and peppercorns. Add any additional fat-burning spices. Add enough filtered water to cover everything by 1 inch.

If using a stockpot, bring the water to a simmer over medium heat, then reduce the heat to low. Cover and let simmer for at least 4 hours and up to 8 hours, adding filtered was as needed so the bones are always covered.

In a slow cooker, cover and cook on low for 8 hours, adding filtered water only if needed so the bones are always covered.

In a pressure cooker or Instant Pot, using your cooker's instructions, bring to full pressure. Reduce the heat to low, maintaining full pressure, and cook for 2 hours. Allow the pressure to naturally release.

When the broth is done, strain it through a fine-mesh strainer. Discard the bones and vegetables, and reserve the meat for another use. (Or you can refrigerate or freeze the bones and reuse them to make another batch of broth.)

Set the broth aside to cool, then cover and refrigerate. When chilled, the broth should be very gelatinous. The broth will keep in the refrigerator for up to 5 days or in the freezer for 3 months or more.

"Broth Loading" Recipes

BEEF OR CHICKEN VEGETABLE SOUP

PREP TIME: **15 MIN.** | COOK TIME: **25 MIN.** | YIELD: **4 TO 6 SERVINGS**

FOR BEEF VEGETABLE SOUP

- 2 tablespoons avocado oil or coconut oil
- 2 garlic cloves, minced
- 1 small onion, diced
- 1 cup diced celery (about 2 ribs)
- 4 cups (1 quart) Beef Bone Broth (page 95)
- 1 (28-ounce) can diced tomatoes
- 1 cup 1-inch pieces green beans
- 1 cup thinly sliced green cabbage (about $1/4$ head)
- 1 cup $1/2$-inch pieces yellow summer squash
- 2 teaspoons Italian seasoning
- 1 teaspoon Celtic or pink Himalayan salt
- $1/2$ teaspoon freshly ground black pepper

FOR CHICKEN VEGETABLE SOUP

- 2 tablespoons avocado oil or coconut oil
- 2 garlic cloves, minced
- 1 small onion, diced
- 1 cup diced celery (about 2 ribs)
- 6 cups ($1^1/2$ quarts) Chicken Bone Broth (page 96)
- 1 cup 1-inch pieces green beans
- 1 cup thinly sliced green cabbage (about $1/4$ head)
- 1 cup ½-inch pieces yellow summer squash
- 2 cups lightly packed baby spinach
- 1 to $1^1/2$ teaspoons dried thyme
- 1 teaspoon Celtic or pink Himalayan salt
- $1/2$ teaspoon freshly ground black pepper

In a large stockpot, heat the oil over medium-high heat. Add the garlic, onion, and celery and reduce the heat to medium-low. Cook, stirring, for 6 to 8 minutes, until softened.

Raise the heat to medium-high and add the broth and all the remaining ingredients. Bring the soup to a simmer, then reduce the heat to medium-low and simmer for 15 to 20 minutes. Serve warm.

CHILLED CUCUMBER SOUP

PREP TIME: **15 MIN.** | COOK TIME: **12 MIN.** | YIELD: **4 TO 6 SERVINGS**

1 cup water

4 medium cucumbers, peeled, seeded, and sliced

1/2 cup sliced yellow onion

1 teaspoon Celtic or pink Himalayan salt

1/2 teaspoon freshly ground black pepper

4 cups (1 quart) Chicken Bone Broth (page 96)

1/2 teaspoon arrowroot powder, blended with 1 teaspoon water

1 small bay leaf

1 cup unsweetened plain almond milk

1 teaspoon minced fresh dill

1 teaspoon minced fresh Italian parsley

1 teaspoon minced fresh chives

1/2 teaspoon lemon zest

Bring the water to a boil over medium-high heat. Add the cucumbers, onion, salt, and pepper and cover. Simmer for 5 to 7 minutes, until the vegetables are very soft.

Purée using a food processor, blender, or immersion blender until smooth. In a large stockpot, bring the bone broth to a simmer and add the arrowroot mixture, bay leaf, and puréed cucumbers. Reduce the heat to low and simmer, stirring for 5 minutes, until the soup thickens.

Let the soup cool to room temperature and add the almond milk, fresh herbs, and lemon zest. Refrigerate. Serve the soup very cold.

NOTE: Use caution when puréeing hot soup in a blender or food processor. Work in small batches and cover the top of the sealed blender or processor with a kitchen towel to avoid getting burned.

CAULIFLOWER VICHYSSOISE

PREP TIME: **15 MIN.** | COOK TIME: **25 MIN.** | YIELD: **4 TO 6 SERVINGS**

2 tablespoons ghee (page 147)

1 garlic clove, minced

2 leeks, white and pale green parts only, cut into thin rounds

4 cups (1 quart) Chicken Bone Broth (page 96)

1/2 cup canned full-fat coconut milk

3 cups cauliflower florets

1/2 teaspoon dried thyme

1 teaspoon Celtic or pink Himalayan salt

1/2 teaspoon freshly ground black pepper, plus more for serving

1/2 teaspoon arrowroot powder, blended with 1 tablespoon water, plus more if needed

In a large stockpot, melt the ghee over medium-high heat. Add the garlic and leeks and reduce the heat to medium-low. Cook, stirring, for 6 to 8 minutes, until softened.

Raise the heat to medium-high and add the broth, coconut milk, cauliflower, thyme, salt, and pepper. When the soup begins to simmer, reduce the heat to medium-low and simmer for 15 to 20 minutes, until the cauliflower is cooked through.

Purée with an immersion blender, blender, or food processor until smooth and creamy. Return to the stockpot and stir in the arrowroot mixture. Simmer for 3 to 5 minutes, until the soup thickens, adding more arrowroot if a thicker soup is desired. Serve warm, garnished with freshly ground black pepper.

CREAMY BROCCOLI SOUP

PREP TIME: **15 MIN.** | COOK TIME: **25 MIN.** | YIELD: **4 TO 6 SERVINGS**

2 tablespoons ghee (page 147)

2 garlic cloves, minced

1 small onion, diced

4 cups (1 quart) Chicken Bone Broth (page 96)

1 cup canned full-fat coconut milk

4 cups broccoli florets

1/2 teaspoon ground nutmeg

1 teaspoon Celtic or pink Himalayan salt

1/2 teaspoon freshly ground black pepper

In a large stockpot, melt the ghee over medium-high heat. Add the garlic and onion and reduce the heat to medium-low. Cook, stirring, for 6 to 8 minutes, until softened.

Raise the heat to medium-high and add the broth, coconut milk, broccoli, nutmeg, salt, and pepper. When the soup begins to boil, reduce the heat to medium-low and simmer for 15 to 20 minutes, until the broccoli is cooked through.

Purée with an immersion blender, blender, or food processor until smooth and creamy. Serve warm.

NOTE: Use caution when puréeing hot soup in a blender or food processor. Work in small batches and cover the top of the sealed blender or processor with a kitchen towel to avoid getting burned.

IS YOUR THYROID MAKING YOUR BELLY FAT?

IZABELLA WENTZ, PHARM D, FASCP

Pharmacist, patient advocate, and #1 *New York Times* bestselling author of *Hashimoto's Protocol: A 90-Day Plan for Reversing Thyroid Symptoms and Getting Your Life Back* and *Hashimoto's Thyroiditis: Lifestyle Interventions for Finding and Treating the Root Cause*

thyroidpharmacist.com

Many people who struggle with their weight have the common thyroid condition known as Hashimoto's thyroiditis. This condition sounds rare and exotic, yet it is present in up to 28% of our population, affecting five to eight women for every man affected. Sadly, most people who have the condition don't even know they have it.

Hashimoto's thyroiditis is an autoimmune condition that results in the destruction of the thyroid gland, eventually leading to hypothyroidism, or an underactive thyroid. Most people with Hashimoto's have a hard time keeping weight off despite maintaining the same diet and exercise routines they have had for years.

This is because the thyroid gland controls our metabolism, and even a slight deficiency in thyroid hormones, such as that caused by an immune-system attack, can slow down metabolism.

Most doctors tell thyroid patients that they simply need to eat less and exercise more. However, this advice can be quite detrimental and put the person's body into a deeper fat-storing mode!

Unfortunately, due to improper testing, most patients are also unaware that they have thyroid disease. Most doctors only test patients using a TSH (thyroid-stimulating hormone) blood test. However, this can lead to many missed diagnoses, because the TSH result can remain normal for as long as a decade while the thyroid gland is under attack by the immune system. Thyroid antibody tests are more accurate and can reveal the metabolism-altering attack on the thyroid gland. I recommend a complete thyroid panel consisting of the following tests: TSH, free T3, free T4, thyroid peroxidase antibodies, thyroglobulin antibodies, and reverse T3.

If you already know that you have a thyroid condition and/or are taking thyroid hormone medications yet are still struggling with your weight, energy level, skin, hair, or mood, I recommend a further investigation into optimizing your hormones, nutrition, gut health, adrenal health, and liver health and addressing your underlying triggers for flare-ups.

1. OPTIMIZING HORMONES

Synthetic thyroid hormone (known as Synthroid or Levothyroxine) is one of the top-selling drugs in the United States; however, there are other thyroid medications that may be more effective. Synthroid contains one of the thyroid hormones, known as T4, while the hormone with the most impact on weight is T3. T4 is a precursor to T3—which means that T3 is formed from T4—but some individuals do not convert T4 to T3 properly. Women with thyroid conditions report more weight loss with T4/T3 combination medications (such as Armour Thyroid, Nature-Throid, or compounded medications) versus T4 medications alone.

2. NUTRITION

While most doctors only look at calories in and calories out, I've found that this approach can be very detrimental to both health and weight loss. In my research involving more than two thousand people with thyroid disease, I've found that nutrient-dense diets free of problematic foods help people with thyroid disease feel better, lose weight, and even reduce their markers of autoimmune disorder. Gluten, dairy, and soy are the most commonly problematic foods in thyroid disease, with 88%, 80%, and 65%, respectively, of thyroid patients reporting feeling better when these foods are removed from their diet.

3. GUT HEALTH

Thyroid disease is intimately connected to gut health. I love recommending bone broth, fermented foods, and probiotics to help with resolving gut issues. New research is showing that people who are overweight have an imbalance of bacterial flora in their guts. The particular bacteria found in overweight people extract more calories from food than the bacteria of people who have a normal weight. This means you could be eating the same amount of food as your skinny friends and gaining more weight from it! Probiotics and fermented foods that contain beneficial bacteria may be helpful with balancing your bacterial flora.

Additional triggers—such as toxins, an impaired stress response, chronic infections, and nutrient deficiencies—can contribute to thyroid disease and weight-loss resistance. For more information on a ninety-day plan that has helped thousands of people already, please check out my book *Hashimoto's Protocol: A 90-Day Plan for Reversing Thyroid Symptoms and Getting Your Life Back.*

ROASTED RED BELL PEPPER SOUP

PREP TIME: **15 MIN.** | COOK TIME: **25 MIN.** | YIELD: **4 TO 6 SERVINGS**

2 tablespoons coconut oil or avocado oil

2 garlic cloves, minced

1 small onion, diced

4 cups (1 quart) Chicken Bone Broth (page 96)

1/2 cup canned full-fat coconut milk

2 cups jarred roasted red peppers, puréed in a blender or food processor

3 cups roughly chopped chard or baby spinach

1/2 cup fresh basil leaves, roughly chopped

1 teaspoon Celtic or pink Himalayan salt

1/2 teaspoon freshly ground black pepper

In a large stockpot, heat the oil over medium-high heat. Add the garlic and onion and reduce the heat to medium-low. Cook, stirring, for 6 to 8 minutes, until softened. Increase the heat to medium-high and add the broth, coconut milk, and puréed peppers.

When the mixture begins to boil, reduce the heat to medium-low and simmer for 15 to 20 minutes. Add the chard, basil, salt, and pepper and simmer for another 3 to 5 minutes. Serve warm.

CREAMY TOMATO FLORENTINE SOUP

PREP TIME: **15 MIN.** | COOK TIME: **25 MIN.** | YIELD: **4 TO 6 SERVINGS**

4 cups (1 quart) Chicken Bone Broth (page 96)

1 (28-ounce) can diced tomatoes

1 garlic clove, smashed

1/2 cup canned full-fat coconut milk

2 teaspoons Italian seasoning

3 cups or more loosely packed baby spinach

1 cup fresh basil leaves, cut into fine ribbons

1 teaspoon Celtic or pink Himalayan salt

1/2 teaspoon freshly ground black pepper

In a large stockpot, heat the broth over medium-high heat. Put the canned tomatoes into a blender and purée until smooth. Add the tomatoes and garlic to the broth and bring to a simmer. Add the coconut milk and Italian seasoning and reduce the heat to medium-low or low. Simmer for 15 to 20 minutes. Add the spinach, basil, salt, and pepper and simmer for another 3 minutes. Serve warm.

PHO

PREP TIME: **15 MIN.** | COOK TIME: **20 MIN** | YIELD: **4 TO 6 SERVINGS**

2 tablespoons avocado oil or coconut oil

2 garlic cloves, minced

3 scallions, cut into 1/2-inch pieces

5 slices fresh ginger

4 cups (1 quart) Beef (page 95) or Chicken Bone Broth (page 96)

1 cup roughly chopped bok choy

1 cup sliced mushrooms

2 tablespoons coconut aminos

1/2 teaspoon Celtic or pink Himalayan salt

1/2 teaspoon freshly ground black or white pepper

Dash of cayenne pepper

2 cups zoodles (about 2 medium zucchini, spiralized; see Note)

1/2 cup fresh cilantro leaves

FOR SERVING (OPTIONAL)

Thai basil

Sriracha sauce

Mung bean sprouts

Lime wedges

In a large stockpot, heat the oil over medium-high heat. Add the garlic, scallions, and ginger and reduce the heat to medium-low. Cook, stirring, for 3 to 4 minutes to soften the scallions. Raise the heat to medium-high and add the broth, bok choy, mushrooms, coconut aminos, salt, black pepper, and cayenne. When the soup begins to boil, reduce the heat to medium-low and simmer for 10 to 15 minutes. Add the zoodles and cilantro and remove from the heat. Serve warm, with Thai basil, sriracha, mung bean sprouts, and lime wedges, if desired.

NOTES: Stores have begun selling precut zoodles to save you time in the kitchen. If you don't have a spiralizer, there are other methods you can use to make zucchini pasta. You can use a julienne peeler to get straight, skinny zoodles. A mandoline or an old-fashioned vegetable peeler will give you wide, flat zoodles.

IS ADRENAL FATIGUE PACKING POUNDS ONTO YOUR BELLY?

There's a good chance you haven't thought about your adrenal glands since high school biology class.

However, if you want to keep belly fat off, you should know what these glands do for you—and how a condition called *adrenal fatigue* can send them into a tailspin, making you miserable and adding inches to your belly.

Here's a quick refresher. Your adrenals are two small glands that sit on top of your kidneys, a little like mushroom caps. These glands have lots of important jobs, and one is to step in when you're stressed and tell your body how to react. When your brain sends danger signals to your adrenals, they respond by cranking out adrenaline, norepinephrine, and cortisol to prepare you for a fight-or-flight reaction.

This job sounds tough enough, but that's not all your adrenal glands do. They also produce a host of other hormones that affect every cell in your body. In particular, they play a big role in producing your sex hormones—and if you're a woman, they pick up the slack in making these hormones as you hit perimenopause and your ovaries produce less of them.

So far, so good. But here's the problem. Your adrenal glands are designed to handle the *acute* stresses that our ancient ancestors faced—for instance, being chased by a lion—but not the *chronic* stress we face today. While these glands can deal brilliantly with brief bouts of stress, they need downtime to get back to normal. And in today's world, there's no downtime. We're constantly under low-level stress, brought on by everything from job pressures to money worries to family crises to traffic and noise.

Under siege from this chronic stress, our adrenal glands crank out cortisol constantly. They're overworked, and eventually they "burn out," giving rise to adrenal fatigue. They no longer produce enough hormones, and they no longer keep these hormones balanced. As a result, you pack on pounds . . . and you feel moody and tired and get a "cortisol tire" around your waist.

What's the solution?

Obviously, getting your stress under control is the best way to prevent or cure adrenal fatigue. In Chapter 10, I serve up some powerful ways to tame that stress.

And here's another key: a healthy diet that's loaded with powerful healing foods—in particular, bone broth. Here's what this "liquid gold" does for your adrenal glands:

- Bone broth supplies a rich dose of *conditional amino acids*—glycine, proline, arginine, and glutamine—which your adrenal glands need to heal themselves. These are amino acids that your body can't supply in adequate quantities if it's run-down.

- The glycine and magnesium in bone broth are calming nutrients that help ease your anxiety.

- Bone broth is loaded with gelatin, which helps to heal that permeable intestine (or *leaky gut*) I talked about in Chapter 1. A leaky gut, which allows toxins to escape into your bloodstream, leads to chronic, system-wide inflammation—and this raises your cortisol levels, contributing to adrenal fatigue. Bone broth soothes your gut and helps make it rock-solid, getting your inflammation under control.

So now you have another reason to drink bone broth every day, even after you finish your 10-Day Belly Slimdown: It'll make your adrenal glands happy, and that in turn can keep a "cortisol tire" at bay!

SPICY MEXICAN SOUP

PREP TIME: **15 MIN.** | COOK TIME: **25 MIN.** | YIELD: **4 TO 6 SERVINGS**

2 tablespoons avocado oil or coconut oil

2 garlic cloves, minced

1 small onion, diced

1 cup diced celery (about 2 ribs)

1 red bell pepper, seeded and diced

4 cups (1 quart) Chicken Bone Broth (page 96)

1 (14.5-ounce) can diced tomatoes

3 cups thinly sliced green cabbage (about ¼ medium head)

1/2 cup fresh cilantro leaves, roughly chopped

1 teaspoon ground cumin

2 to 3 teaspoons chili powder

1/2 teaspoon dried oregano

Dash of cayenne pepper

1 teaspoon Celtic or pink Himalayan salt

1/2 teaspoon freshly ground black pepper

1 small jalapeño, sliced, for serving (optional)

Lime wedges, for serving (optional)

In a large stockpot, heat the oil over medium-high heat. Add the garlic, onion, celery, and bell pepper and reduce the heat to medium-low. Cook, stirring, for 6 to 8 minutes, until softened.

Increase the heat to medium-high and add the remaining ingredients except the jalapeño and lime wedges. When the soup begins to boil, reduce the heat to medium-low and simmer for 15 to 20 minutes. Serve warm, with jalapeño slices and lime wedges, if desired.

BONE BROTH AND THE GLUTAMINE ISSUE

I love bone broth because it's loaded with nutrients that heal your gut, erase your wrinkles, soothe your joints, and blast your belly fat. But it also contains one nutrient that can give a few people some trouble at first. That nutrient is *glutamine*—and I want to talk about it with you.

First, here's a little background. Glutamine is an amino acid that plays lots of roles in your body. You need glutamine to keep your immune system healthy, to help you recover from wounds and illnesses, and to build your muscles. It's also critical for healthy digestion and brain function.

And here's something else to know: Even if you aren't

drinking bone broth, your diet (if it's healthy) is high in glutamine. Meat, chicken, and fish are rich in it. So are such veggies as spinach and cabbage. (Breast milk is a rich source of glutamine, too, showing that Mother Nature wants infants to get plenty of this nutrient, as well.)

So glutamine is already a part of your diet—and it's a good guy. However . . .

Some people can't metabolize glutamine well. This problem can stem from a variety of causes, including a severely sick gut, lead toxicity, a deficiency of vitamin B_6, or overexposure to monosodium glutamate (MSG). People who have issues with glutamine may find that upping their intake of this nutrient upsets their stomach, gives them headaches, or makes them feel tired or "foggy."

Luckily, if you've been diagnosed with this problem, there's a simple solution. Initially, instead of drinking bone broth, switch to *meat* broth. This is broth you make by simmering bone-in cuts of beef, lamb, or poultry. (Don't remove the bones from the meat.) Because you simmer meat broth for only a few hours—two hours or so for poultry, four hours or so for beef or lamb—it has a much lower glutamine content than long-simmered bone broth.

Once you detoxify your cells, give your body the nutrients it needs, and build a strong gut wall, you'll be able to benefit from the healing power of bone broth. After a few weeks of drinking meat broth, start adding bone broth into your diet gradually. At first, try very small amounts— maybe 1/4 cup—and increase the amount every few days. If you have any problems, go back to drinking meat broth.

And here's another tip: Skim the fat from your broth after it cools. Some people who *think* they have an issue with glutamine actually have difficulty digesting the fat in bone broth.

Try these two simple tricks—switching temporarily to meat broth, and skimming the fat from your broth—and see what happens. Odds are, you and bone broth will be the best of buddies in just a few weeks!

WATERCRESS SOUP

PREP TIME: **10 MIN.** | COOK TIME: **10 MIN.** | YIELD: **4 TO 6 SERVINGS**

2 tablespoons ghee (page 147) or pastured butter

1 medium onion, diced

2 garlic cloves, minced

4 cups (1 quart) Chicken Bone Broth (page 96)

1/2 to 1 teaspoon Celtic or pink Himalayan salt

1/2 teaspoon freshly ground black or white pepper

1/2 cup canned full-fat coconut milk (optional, for a creamier soup)

2 bunches of watercress (about 14 ounces), thick stems removed

In a large stockpot, melt the ghee over medium-high heat. Add the onion and garlic, reduce the heat to medium-low, and cook, stirring, for 6 to 8 minutes, until softened.

Raise the heat to medium-high and add the broth, salt, and pepper. If using the coconut milk, add it now. Bring to a boil, then reduce the heat to medium-low and simmer for 3 minutes. Add the watercress and simmer for about 1 minute, just to wilt the watercress. Watercress soup can be served as is or puréed. Purée with an immersion blender, blender, or food processor until smooth and creamy.

NOTE: Use caution when puréeing hot soup in a blender or food processor. Work in small batches, and cover the top of the sealed blender or processor with a kitchen towel to avoid getting burned.

DRESS IT UP WITH DIVINE CONDIMENTS

B y now you know I'm ruthless about taking those extra pounds off you. No grains, no sugar, no dairy, no soy, no junk. No exceptions. No excuses.

Well, guess what—now I'm going to lay down yet another law. Here it is: You must use *no unapproved condiments*. That includes just about all commercial versions of mayonnaise, ketchup, and salad dressings.

This is one of those times when I know you might be tempted to cheat. After all, you're thinking, "Seriously . . . how much damage can a teeny-tiny spoonful of ranch dressing, ketchup, or mayo really do?"

Unfortunately, the answer is . . . a lot.

Face it: The condiments you get at the grocery store are mostly just *awful*. If you doubt me, go to your fridge right now and pull out random bottles. Now read the ingredient lists on the back of them.

Even if you're using the top brands, you'll see such ingredients as artificial colors, MSG, partially hydrogenated soybean oil, high-fructose corn syrup, gluten, cornstarch, emulsifiers, and fillers. Just reading the label on your ranch dressing may give you a heart attack—never mind actually eating it.

If you're still reluctant to give up your favorite condiments, let me offer you a little more incentive. Here's a look at just some of the damage the additives in condiments can do to you:

- Food companies use additives called *emulsifiers* to blend ingredients together. Often, condiments are loaded with synthetic emulsifiers. In one recent experiment, scientists fed two of them—with the yummy names of polysorbate-80 and carboxymethylcellulose—to mice. The result: The mice got fat and sick.[1]

- Many condiments are swimming in high-fructose corn syrup (HFCS). HFCS is a real belly-fat bad boy, packing fat onto you even faster than sugar does. One researcher studying its effects on rats said, "These rats aren't just getting fat; they're demonstrating characteristics of obesity, including substantial increases in abdominal fat and circulating triglycerides."[2]

- MSG, found in hundreds of condiments, is an *excitotoxin* that overstimulates your brain, causing it to produce too much dopamine.

- Certain condiment additives, when mixed together, can act synergistically to damage your brain cells.[3]

Ounce for ounce, commercial condiments are one of the worst food groups in the world when it comes to making you fat and sick. The sugars and other unhealthy additives in them are so concentrated that even a teaspoon or two can lead to an additive overdose.

Luckily, I have good news: It's far easier than you think to make your own condiments and salad dressings. You don't need to be an Iron Chef to do it; you just need a few minutes and a good recipe. What's more, you're going to *love* how much better the do-it-yourself versions are than that stale, additive-loaded stuff in a bottle.

In this chapter, I'll show you how to dress up your 10-Day Belly Slimdown meals with creamy mayo, tangy vinaigrettes, and ranch dressing for salads or dipping. Each recipe is yummy, and trust me: You'll never miss all those additives!

10-Day Belly Slimdown Condiments and Salad Dressings

AVOCADO OIL MAYONNAISE

PREP TIME: **15 MIN.** | YIELD: **A LITTLE OVER 1 CUP** | 1 TABLESPOON = 1 FAT SERVING

2 large egg yolks

1/2 teaspoon dry mustard

1/2 teaspoon Dijon mustard

2 tablespoons fresh lemon juice

1/2 teaspoon Celtic or pink Himalayan salt

1 cup avocado oil

Stevia or monk fruit sweetener, to equal 1/4 teaspoon sugar (optional)

Bring all the ingredients to room temperature. Put the egg yolks in a food processor or blender. Add both mustards, the lemon juice, and the salt. Pulse until combined.

With the motor running, add the oil in a *very, very slow and steady stream*. The mixture should become thick and emulsified. Add the sweetener, if using. Refrigerate in an airtight container for up to 5 days.

NOTES: Use yolks from very fresh, organic, free-range eggs with un-cracked shells or use pasteurized eggs. If you've ever tried to make mayonnaise, you may have experienced a failure in which the product does not emulsify or completely combine to form a silky end product. Adding the lemon juice should help, but the real trick is the *slow, slow, slow* stream of oil while blending. The stream of oil should look as fine as a thread as you pour. Take a full 3 minutes to add the oil.

DAIRY-FREE CREAMY RANCH DRESSING

PREP TIME: **10 MIN.** | YIELD: **A LITTLE OVER 1 CUP** | 2 TABLESPOONS = 1 FAT SERVING

1/2 cup Avocado Oil Mayonnaise (page 117)

1 teaspoon fresh thyme leaves

1 or 2 garlic cloves, smashed

1/4 cup roughly chopped chives

1 tablespoon roughly chopped fresh dill

2 tablespoons roughly chopped fresh Italian parsley leaves

1/2 cup full-fat coconut milk

1 tablespoon white wine vinegar or champagne vinegar

1/2 teaspoon dry mustard

Celtic or pink Himalayan salt

Freshly ground black pepper

In a food processor, combine the mayonnaise, thyme, garlic, chives, dill, and parsley and process until the herbs are chopped.

With the motor running, slowly pour in the coconut milk and then add the vinegar, mustard, and salt and pepper to taste. Taste and adjust the seasoning. Transfer to a jar or airtight container and refrigerate for up to 2 weeks.

VARIATIONS

You can also use dried herbs if you choose. When herbs are dried, their aromatic oils are concentrated. As a general rule of thumb, use about one-third as much dried herbs as fresh herbs. If the recipe calls for 1 tablespoon of a fresh herb, use about 1 teaspoon dried, but always taste and adjust to your liking. If the dried herbs have been in your pantry for a year or more, they have lost much of their potency, so it's time to replace them.

If you like the flavor of smoky chipotle, you can make a Chipotle Ranch Dressing by adding 1 (or 2, if you're daring) canned chipotles in adobo sauce.

COMMERCIAL CONDIMENTS THAT PASS MY TOUGH TEST

While most commercial condiments are dreadful, you can find versions that are superhealthy if you're willing to look for them. Here are three of the best:

Salsa. It's easy to find fresh, additive-free salsas at a regular supermarket these days. You can also find additive-free jarred versions at health food stores.

Avocado mayo. As the demand for this condiment sky-rockets, more and more stores now carry it. (For instance, Costco carries Chosen Foods avocado mayo, and a growing number of stores carry Primal Kitchen Mayo.) You can also buy avocado mayo online.

Mustard. This is one condiment that manufacturers actually get right much of the time. Read the labels, and make sure all the ingredients are clean and natural.

Happily, more and more healthy, low-carb condiments are joining this list. Primal Kitchen, for instance, now offers a line of salad dressings and marinades, as well as a good-for-you ketchup.

SWEET VIDALIA ONION VINAIGRETTE

PREP TIME: **10 MIN.** | YIELD: **ABOUT 1 CUP** | 2 TABLESPOONS = 1 FAT SERVING

- 1/2 cup chopped Vidalia or other sweet onion
- 1/4 cup champagne vinegar or white wine vinegar
- 1 teaspoon dry mustard
- 1/2 cup olive oil
- 1/2 teaspoon Celtic or pink Himalayan salt
- 2 teaspoons poppy seeds
- Stevia or monk fruit sweetener to equal 2 to 3 teaspoons sugar, or to taste

In a blender, combine the onion, vinegar, mustard, oil, and salt and blend until smooth. Transfer to a jar or airtight container, add the poppy seeds, and taste. Add the sweetener gradually to your liking. Cover and refrigerate for up to 5 days.

KIMCHI

PREP TIME: **30 MIN. (ACTIVE)** | YIELD: **ABOUT 4 CUPS**

1 medium head napa cabbage

1/4 cup Celtic or pink Himalayan salt (do not use iodized salt)

Filtered, nonchlorinated water

5 garlic cloves, grated or minced

1 teaspoon grated fresh ginger (about 1/2-inch knob)

2 tablespoons fish sauce or water

1 to 5 tablespoons Korean red pepper flakes (*gochugaru*; see Notes)

3/4 cup peeled daikon matchsticks

4 scallions, cut into 1-inch pieces

2 carrots, cut into matchsticks

Wash the cabbage, cut it lengthwise into 2-inch-thick slices, and discard the center core. Put the cabbage in a large bowl and add the salt. Massage with your hands for a few minutes until it starts to soften, cover with filtered water, place a plate on top of the cabbage, and weight the plate down with something heavy, such as a can of tomatoes. Let stand at room temperature for about 1 1/2 hours.

Put the cabbage in a colander and rinse well at least three times. Set aside to drain for 15 minutes while you make the seasoning paste.

In a large bowl, combine the garlic, ginger, fish sauce or water, and Korean red pepper flakes to make a paste. Add the daikon, scallions, and carrots. Squeeze out any moisture left in the cabbage and combine it with the other vegetables and spicy paste. Wearing rubber gloves, gently mix all the ingredients together and pack into a clean glass jar until the liquid rises above the vegetables. Leaving at least 1 to 2 inches of headroom, loosely seal the jar, and put it on a plate or in a bowl to collect any juices that overflow while the kimchi ferments. Keep the mixture at room temperature so the vegetables can ferment; do not refrigerate.

Open the jar once daily to pack down the vegetables using a clean utensil and allow the gases produced during fermentation to be released. This is also the time to taste it to see if it is fermented to your liking. After tasting, do NOT insert the utensil back into the kimchi. You will likely want 2 to 4 days of fermentation, unless you're a hard-core kimchi fan. The longer it ferments, the stronger it gets. When done, refrigerate. Serve immediately or store in the refrigerator for 1 to 2 weeks.

NOTES: Fermented foods heal the gut by feeding it healthy bacteria.

Korean red pepper flakes, or *gochugaru,* is a sun-dried Korean chile pepper that has been ground to a flaky/powdery texture. You can find it online or in Asian groceries. It is very hot and spicy with a bit of smokiness. Use 1 to 5 tablespoons depending on how hot you like your kimchi; if you are making it for the first time, start with about 2 tablespoons.

TOMATO VINAIGRETTE

PREP TIME: **10 MIN.** | YIELD: **ABOUT 1 CUP** | 2 TABLESPOONS = 1 FAT SERVING

1/2 cup chopped ripe tomatoes

1/2 cup packed roughly chopped fresh basil

2 tablespoons minced sweet onion

1/4 cup red wine vinegar

1/2 cup olive oil

1/2 teaspoon Celtic or pink Himalayan salt

Freshly ground black pepper

Stevia or monk fruit sweetener (optional)

1 garlic clove, smashed

Combine the tomatoes, basil, onion, and vinegar in a blender or food processor and blend until smooth. With the machine running, add the oil in a slow stream and process until well blended. Season with the salt, and pepper and sweetener (if using) to taste. Transfer to a jar or airtight container and add the garlic. Cover and refrigerate for up to 5 days.

GET IT DONE WITH FAT-BUSTING SHAKES

What's better than a rich, creamy, ice-cold shake from your favorite fast-food joint? A shake that's actually *good* for you . . . and melts your belly fat, too!

On the 10-Day Belly Slimdown, you're going to indulge in a smooth, delicious shake every single day. And you're going to burn belly fat at the same time.

What's the secret? Simply replace that unhealthy ice cream with beautiful, clean protein or collagen powder in a flavor you love—chocolate, vanilla, coffee, or maybe even orange. Add a little natural sweetness from blueberries, monk fruit sweetener, or stevia if you like.

Next, toss in two handfuls of your favorite leafy greens. Spinach is one of my top choices because it adds satisfying fiber without changing the taste of your shake. Add a dose of healthy fat, which will give your shake that creamy consistency you crave, and you have a cool, sweet drink that will transport you back to your childhood as it melts your belly fat off you.

In this chapter, you'll find eleven variations on a basic shake, all delicious and all packed with fat-burning power. You can have a different shake every day or repeat your favorites—it's totally up to you. Enjoy!

10-Day Belly Slimdown Shake Recipes

BELLY-BUSTING SHAKE

PREP TIME: **10 MIN.** | YIELD: **1 SERVING**

This unique recipe was contributed by my friend Karen Pickus, chef and food stylist at Good Morning America, *who's a big fan of healthy shakes.*

1/2 cup loosely packed baby kale leaves

1 small Persian cucumber, or 1/2 regular cucumber, unpeeled

12 fresh mint leaves

1/4 teaspoon mild curry powder

2 dashes of ground cinnamon

1 dash of cayenne pepper (optional)

1/2 cup canned full-fat coconut milk

1/2 cup water

1 scoop Dr. Kellyann's Vanilla Bone Broth Protein Powder or vanilla beef protein (15 to 25 grams protein)

3 ice cubes

Place all the ingredients in a blender. Blend for 1 minute and serve.

Recipe courtesy Karen Pickus 2017 • Recipe developed and written by Karen Pickus 2017

BERRY SHAKE

PREP TIME: **3 MIN.** | YIELD: **1 SERVING**

1 cup water, unsweetened carrageenan-free almond milk, or unsweetened coconut milk (not canned)

1 scoop Dr. Kellyann's Vanilla Bone Broth Protein Powder or vanilla beef protein (15 to 25 grams protein)

Handful of fresh or frozen blueberries

$1/2$ teaspoon pure vanilla extract (optional)

2 handfuls of leafy greens (watercress, kale, spinach, Swiss chard, etc.)

1 tablespoon coconut oil

Ice (optional; add to blender or pour shake over ice)

Monk fruit sweetener or stevia for additional sweetness (optional)

Pour the liquids into a blender, then add all the other ingredients. Blend until smooth and serve.

CHOCOLATE ALMOND SHAKE

PREP TIME: **3 MIN.** | YIELD: **1 SERVING**

1 cup water, unsweetened carrageenan-free almond milk, or unsweetened coconut milk (not canned)

1 scoop Dr. Kellyann's Chocolate Bone Broth Protein Powder or chocolate beef protein (15 to 25 grams protein)

2 handfuls of leafy greens (watercress, kale, spinach, Swiss chard, etc.)

1 tablespoon unsweetened almond butter

Ice (optional; add to blender or pour shake over ice)

Monk fruit sweetener or stevia for additional sweetness (optional)

Pour the liquids into a blender, then add all the other ingredients. Blend until smooth and serve.

CHOCOLATE COCONUT SHAKE

PREP TIME: **3 MIN.** | YIELD: **1 SERVING**

1 cup water, unsweetened carrageenan-free almond milk, or unsweetened coconut milk (not canned)

1 scoop Dr. Kellyann's Chocolate Bone Broth Protein Powder or chocolate beef protein (15 to 25 grams protein)

2 handfuls of leafy greens (watercress, kale, spinach, Swiss chard, etc.)

$1/3$ to $1/2$ (14-ounce) can full-fat coconut milk

Ice (optional; add to blender or pour shake over ice)

Monk fruit sweetener or stevia for additional sweetness (optional)

Pour the liquids into a blender, then add all the other ingredients. Blend until smooth and serve.

THICK-AND-CREAMY CHOCOLATE MINT SHAKE

PREP TIME: **3 MIN.** | YIELD: **1 SERVING**

1 cup water, unsweetened carrageenan-free almond milk, or unsweetened coconut milk (not canned)

1 scoop Dr. Kellyann's Chocolate Bone Broth Protein Powder or chocolate beef protein (15 to 25 grams protein)

$1/4$ teaspoon pure mint extract, or a small cluster of fresh mint leaves

2 handfuls of leafy greens (watercress, kale, spinach, Swiss chard, etc.)

$1/4$ to $1/2$ avocado

Ice (optional; add to blender or pour shake over ice)

Monk fruit sweetener or stevia for additional sweetness (optional)

Pour the liquids into a blender, then add all the other ingredients. Blend until smooth and serve.

SAY "YES" TO WHEY!

If you've read any of my earlier books, you may remember that I used to say no to whey protein powder. But now I've done a complete 180 on this.

Why? Because I'm open-minded, and sometimes I discover that a food I've put on my "no list" deserves to move over to the "yes list." And that's what I've decided about whey protein—but *only* the right form of this protein. Here's the story.

If you know me, you know I'm not a fan of dairy. I can't tolerate most dairy foods, and neither can my patients. I estimate that about 80 percent of people have issues with dairy—for instance, gas, bloating, and blotchy skin—and most of them don't even know it. So why am I moving whey isolate to my yes list? After all, it's a dairy product, because it's a combination of proteins isolated from whey, the liquid part of milk that separates during cheese production.

Here are my reasons. When it comes to dairy sensitivity, whey typically isn't the issue. Instead, it's lactose. Whey protein isolate is lactose-free, because unlike whey protein concentrate—another common form of whey protein—it undergoes extra purification to remove the lactose. Simply look for the word *isolate* on the label, and you'll know you're getting the right stuff (and *only* the right stuff).

And here's great news: the amino acids in whey protein isolate can help you build muscle and fight sarcopenia, or age-related muscle wasting. In addition, whey is rich in other health-promoting nutrients that can enhance immune function,[2] lower high blood pressure,[3] and lower fasting insulin levels in overweight people.[4]

So if you've been shunning whey protein, now's the time to give it a try. Just make sure you reach for *whey protein isolate*, and you're good to go.

COCONUT MATCHA SHAKE

PREP TIME: **3 MIN.** | YIELD: **1 SERVING**

1 cup water, unsweetened carrageenan-free almond milk, or unsweetened coconut milk (not canned)

1 teaspoon matcha powder (powdered green tea)

1 scoop Dr. Kellyann's Vanilla Bone Broth Protein Powder or vanilla beef protein (15 to 25 grams protein)

2 handfuls of leafy greens (watercress, kale, spinach, Swiss chard, etc.)

1/3 to 1/2 (14-ounce) can full-fat coconut milk

Ice (optional; add to blender or pour shake over ice)

Monk fruit sweetener or stevia for additional sweetness (optional)

Pour the liquids into a blender, then add all the other ingredients. Blend until smooth and serve.

CREAMY ORANGE SHAKE

PREP TIME: **3 MIN.** | YIELD: **1 SERVING**

1 cup water, unsweetened carrageenan-free almond milk, or unsweetened coconut milk (not canned)

1 scoop Dr. Kellyann's Vanilla Bone Broth Protein Powder or vanilla beef protein (15 to 25 grams protein)

1 package Dr. Kellyann's Orange Cream Collagen Cooler or other orange-flavored collagen powder

2 handfuls of leafy greens (watercress, kale, spinach, Swiss chard, etc.)

1 tablespoon avocado oil

Ice (optional; add to blender or pour shake over ice)

Monk fruit sweetener or stevia for additional sweetness (optional)

Pour the liquids into a blender, then add all the other ingredients. Blend until smooth and serve.

"HOT" CHOCOLATE SHAKE

PREP TIME: **3 MIN.** | YIELD: **1 SERVING**

1 cup water, unsweetened carrageenan-free almond milk, or unsweetened coconut milk (not canned)

1 scoop Dr. Kellyann's Chocolate Bone Broth Protein Powder or chocolate beef protein (15 to 25 grams protein)

Pinch or two of ground cinnamon

Pinch of cayenne pepper

Pinch of chili powder (optional)

2 handfuls of leafy greens (watercress, kale, spinach, Swiss chard, etc.)

1 tablespoon avocado oil

Ice (optional; add to blender or pour shake over ice)

Monk fruit sweetener or stevia for additional sweetness (optional)

Pour the liquids into a blender, then add all the other ingredients. Blend until smooth and serve.

LATTE SHAKE

PREP TIME: **3 MIN.** | YIELD: **1 SERVING**

1 cup water, unsweetened carrageenan-free almond milk, or unsweetened coconut milk (not canned)

1 scoop Dr. Kellyann's Chocolate Bone Broth Protein Powder or chocolate beef protein (15 to 25 grams protein)

1 package Collagen Coffee™, or 1/2 teaspoon espresso powder

2 handfuls of leafy greens (watercress, kale, spinach, Swiss chard, etc.)

1 tablespoon coconut oil

Ice (optional; add to blender or pour shake over ice)

Monk fruit sweetener or stevia for additional sweetness (optional)

Pour the liquids into a blender, then add all the other ingredients. Blend until smooth and serve.

WHAT IS MCT OIL?

MCT stands for *medium-chain triglyceride*. MCTs are the cleanest, most direct sources of energy for your body. Your body metabolizes these fatty acids in a different way than it does other fatty acids, increasing the number of calories you burn. Because they're rapidly turned into ketones, MCTs also give your brain a quick shot of energizing fuel that can wake you up in a healthier way than those additive-loaded "energy drinks." In addition, studies show that they're more satiating than other fats.[1]

My favorite MCT oil is David Asprey's Brain Octane Oil. Add a serving of this to your afternoon shake, and you'll take your fat burning to an even higher level!

GINGER SPICE SHAKE

PREP TIME: **10 MIN.** | YIELD: **1 SERVING**

2 whole black peppercorns

1/4 teaspoon ground cinnamon

2 or 3 slices peeled fresh ginger

1 whole clove

1 green tea bag

1 black tea bag

1 scoop Dr. Kellyann's Vanilla Bone Broth Protein Powder or vanilla beef protein (15 to 25 grams protein)

2 handfuls of leafy greens (watercress, kale, spinach, Swiss chard, etc.)

1 tablespoon coconut oil

Ice (optional; add to blender or pour shake over ice)

Monk fruit sweetener or stevia for additional sweetness (optional)

In a small saucepan, combine the peppercorns, cinnamon, ginger, clove, and 1 1/4 cups water. Bring to a boil, then reduce the heat to maintain a simmer, add the tea bags, and let steep for 3 to 5 minutes. Strain the tea through a fine-mesh sieve. Cool. Pour the liquids into the blender first, then add all the other ingredients. Blend until smooth and serve.

VANILLA SPICE SHAKE

PREP TIME: **3 MIN.** | YIELD: **1 SERVING**

1 cup water, unsweetened carrageenan-free almond milk, or unsweetened coconut milk (not canned)

1 scoop Dr. Kellyann's Vanilla Bone Broth Protein Powder or vanilla beef protein (15 to 25 grams protein)

Pinch or two of ground cinnamon

Dash of cayenne pepper

Dash of ground ginger, or 1 slice of peeled fresh ginger

Dash of ground turmeric

Dash of ground nutmeg

2 handfuls of leafy greens (watercress, kale, spinach, Swiss chard, etc.)

2 tablespoons hemp seeds

Ice (optional; add to blender or pour shake over ice)

Monk fruit sweetener or stevia for additional sweetness (optional)

Pour the liquids into a blender, then add all the other ingredients. Blend until smooth and serve.

POWER IT UP WITH SLIM PLATE MEALS

When 7:00 p.m. rolls around each day on your diet, it's time to celebrate. Draw a big red X over that day on your calendar and do your happy dance, because you now have one more day under your belt. Then sit down and savor a full plate of filling, fabulous, fat-burning foods. You've earned it!

What's more, you're now in for a treat. Forget about those bland, boring diet meals you pull out of the microwave. This is a meal you can really look forward to.

That's why I want you to spoil yourself a little. To fully enjoy your dinner, I'd like you to turn it into a special occasion. Set the table with your best dishes, light a candle, and put on some nice music. To make your meal even more festive, mix sparkling water with a slice of cucumber and a squeeze of lemon to make yourself a glass of spa water.

Remember, this isn't tasteless diet food. This is *awesome* food that you're going to love. So kick back and enjoy . . . and pat yourself on the back for another successful day of belly-blasting!

In this chapter, you'll find four sets of recipes. The first set includes proteins you can batch cook for your mini-meals, as well as entrées you can make from those batch-cooked proteins. The second set showcases veggies that will pair beautifully with your proteins. The third section serves up SLIM Plate meals that combine all the ingredients of a mini-meal, while the fourth section features easy, one-pot meals to save on dishwashing!

Proteins

You can batch cook many of these proteins ahead of time (see Chapter 4), then combine them with other ingredients to make quick and easy entrées.

BAKED SALMON

PREP TIME: **5 MIN.** | COOK TIME: **15 TO 25 MIN.** | YIELD: **4 SERVINGS**

1 pound salmon fillet or pieces

1 tablespoon pasture butter or ghee (page 147), melted

Celtic or pink Himalayan salt

Freshly ground black pepper

Small handful of fresh dill, or about 1/2 teaspoon dried dill

1 lemon, cut into thin rounds

Preheat the oven to 400°F and place a rack in the center of the oven.

Tear a long piece of foil, large enough to create a sealed pocket for the salmon. Place the salmon skin-side down on the foil and pour the butter over the fish. Season with salt, pepper, and the dill. Top with the lemon rounds. Carefully wrap the fish in the foil, sealing the edges, and place on a baking sheet.

Bake for 15 minutes and check for doneness. Salmon is done when the meat flakes easily and the fish is opaque on the inside. If needed, reseal and return to the oven until done. Baking time will vary based on your oven, thickness of fish, and the cut (i.e., fillet or pieces).

If you are not eating immediately, let the fish cool completely, package it in individual servings, and refrigerate. Salmon will keep in the refrigerator for 2 to 3 days.

NOTE: Once the salmon is done, you can open the foil and place it under the broiler for 2 to 3 minutes to brown the top, if you like. It can burn quickly, so monitor the broiler.

FAST AND EASY BEEF BURGERS

PREP TIME: **10 MIN.** | COOK TIME: **10 TO 12 MIN.** | YIELD: **4 SERVINGS**

- 1¼ pounds ground beef or ground sirloin
- 1 tablespoon coconut aminos or Worcestershire sauce
- ½ to 1 teaspoon steak seasoning (Montreal steak seasoning works well)
- Salt and freshly ground black pepper

Heat a grill to high or heat a grill pan or skillet over medium-high heat.

Gently combine the beef, coconut aminos, and steak seasoning and form into 4 patties. Season with salt and pepper. Make an indentation in the center of each patty with your thumb so the burgers cook more evenly.

Cook on the grill or in the pan for 5 to 6 minutes per side, depending on thickness, or to an internal temperature of 165°F.

FAST AND EASY TURKEY BURGERS

PREP TIME: **10 MIN.** | COOK TIME: **10 TO 12 MIN.** | YIELD: **4 SERVINGS**

1¼ pounds ground turkey

3 tablespoons minced onion

3 tablespoons finely chopped fresh Italian parsley

½ teaspoon garlic powder

Dash of cayenne pepper

½ to 1 teaspoon Celtic or pink Himalayan salt

¼ to ½ teaspoon freshly ground black pepper

Heat a grill to high or heat a grill pan or skillet over medium-high heat.

Gently combine all the ingredients and form into 4 patties. Make an indentation in the center of each patty with your thumb so the burgers cook more evenly.

Cook on the grill or in the pan for 5 to 6 minutes per side, depending on thickness, or to an internal temperature of 165°F.

ROAST BEEF

PREP TIME: **15 MIN.** | COOK TIME: **45 MIN. TO 8 HRS., DEPENDING ON COOKING METHOD** | YIELD: **6 SERVINGS**

3 to 3½ pounds boneless beef chuck roast, trimmed of excess fat

2 teaspoons Celtic or pink Himalayan salt

1 teaspoon freshly ground black pepper

1 teaspoon garlic powder

1 tablespoon ghee (page 147) or avocado oil

1 large onion, cut into wedges

1 cup Beef (page 95) or Chicken (page 96) Bone Broth, or 1 cup canned puréed tomatoes

Several sprigs of your favorite herbs (I like thyme, bay leaf, and rosemary)

On a cutting board, rub the beef with the salt, pepper, and garlic powder.

In a heavy skillet or Dutch oven, melt the ghee over medium-high heat. Add the beef and brown it on all sides, 5 to 7 minutes per side. Add the onion, broth, and herbs and cover the skillet.

Reduce the heat to low and cook for 3 to 5 hours, until the meat is fork-tender. If needed, add additional broth, water, or puréed tomato as the meat cooks.

To prepare in a slow cooker, brown the meat as directed, put all the ingredients in the slow cooker, cover, and cook on low for 6 to 8 hours. If needed, add additional broth, water, or puréed tomato as the meat cooks.

To prepare in a pressure cooker or Instant Pot, using your cooker's instructions, bring to full pressure. Reduce the heat to low, maintaining full pressure, and cook for 45 minutes. Allow the pressure to naturally release.

The roast can be refrigerated for up to 4 days or frozen for up to 3 months.

ROAST CHICKEN WITH HERBS AND LEMON

PREP TIME: **10 MIN.** | COOK TIME: **50 MIN. TO 1^1/2 HRS.** | YIELD: **6 TO 9 SERVINGS**

1 (3- to 4-pound) whole roasting chicken

^{1}/2 to 1 teaspoon garlic powder

1 teaspoon Celtic or pink Himalayan salt, or to taste

^{1}/2 teaspoon freshly ground black pepper, or to taste

Fresh herbs (rosemary and thyme are a great combination)

1 lemon, cut into wedges

Preheat the oven to 450°F and place a rack in the center of the oven.

Remove the giblets and rinse the cavity and outside of the chicken. Blot the chicken dry inside and out with paper towels and place it in a roasting pan. Generously sprinkle the inside and outside of the chicken with the garlic powder, salt, and pepper, using more or less as desired. Insert the fresh herbs and lemon wedges into the chicken cavity.

Transfer the chicken to the oven and immediately reduce the heat to 400°F. Roast for 50 minutes, checking for doneness by inserting a meat thermometer into the thickest part of the thigh. When done, it should read at least 165°F. If it isn't done, continue roasting and check the temperature every 10 to 15 minutes. Depending on the size of the chicken and your oven, it could take up to 1½ hours.

Let the chicken cool on the counter. Remove the skin and bones, reserving the bones for bone broth. Optionally, package the meat in palm-size portions (approximately 4 to 6 ounces for women, 5 to 8 ounces for men) and refrigerate or freeze. The chicken can be refrigerated for up to 4 days or frozen for up to 3 months.

NOTE: When you roast a whole chicken, you are left with about 60% or a bit more meat calculated by the total raw weight. So if you roasted a 4-pound chicken, your yield will be about 2½ pounds of meat.

SALMON PATTIES

PREP TIME: **15 MIN.** | COOK TIME: **10 MIN.** | YIELD: **4 SERVINGS** | 1 SERVING = 1 FAT

1 large egg

1 teaspoon paprika

2 teaspoons Dijon mustard

1/2 teaspoon Celtic or pink Himalayan salt

1/4 teaspoon freshly ground black pepper

1/2 teaspoon hot sauce

1/2 teaspoon lemon zest

1 pound wild salmon, rinsed, patted dry with paper towels, and diced

1/4 cup finely diced yellow onion

1/4 cup finely diced celery

1 small garlic clove, minced

1/2 cup almond flour

2 tablespoons ghee (page 147) or avocado oil

Lemon wedges, for serving (optional)

In a medium bowl, whisk together the egg, paprika, mustard, salt, pepper, hot sauce, and lemon zest.

In a separate bowl, combine the salmon, onion, celery, garlic, and almond flour. Toss to combine.

Add the salmon mixture to the egg mixture and stir. Form the mixture into 4 patties.

In a large skillet, melt the ghee over medium heat. Cook the patties for 4 to 5 minutes, until golden brown on the first side. Gently turn with an offset spatula and brown the second side for 3 to 4 minutes. Carefully remove the patties from the pan and place on a paper towel to drain.

Serve with lemon wedges, if desired.

SHRIMP CAKES

PREP TIME: **10 MIN.** | COOK TIME: **20 MIN.** | YIELD: **4 SERVINGS** | 1 SERVING = 1 FAT

1 pound raw shrimp, peeled, deveined, and chopped

1/4 red bell pepper, seeded and finely chopped

1 small celery rib, finely chopped

1 garlic clove, minced

2 tablespoons finely chopped red onion

1/2 teaspoon lemon zest

1/2 teaspoon Celtic or pink Himalayan salt

1/4 teaspoon freshly ground black pepper

1 large egg

1/2 cup finely chopped fresh Italian parsley

1/4 cup almond flour

2 tablespoons pastured butter or ghee (page 147)

In a large bowl, combine all the ingredients except the butter. Form into 12 small (2- to 2½-inch-diameter) cakes, each about ½ inch thick.

In a large skillet, melt 1 tablespoon of the butter over medium heat. Very gently place 6 patties into the skillet and cook for 4 to 5 minutes, until the patties begin to turn golden. Very carefully flip the patties using an offset spatula. Cook for 3 to 4 minutes more and place on a paper towel to drain. Melt the remaining 1 tablespoon butter in the pan and repeat with the remaining 6 patties.

SLOW COOKER PULLED PORK

PREP TIME: **10 MIN.** | COOK TIME: **8 HRS.** | YIELD: **6 TO 8 SERVINGS**

2 yellow onions, quartered

1 (3- to 4-pound) pork shoulder

3 garlic cloves, minced, or
1 teaspoon garlic powder

2 teaspoons chili powder

1 teaspoon dried oregano

1 teaspoon ground cumin

Dash of cayenne pepper

1 tablespoon Celtic or pink
Himalayan salt

1 teaspoon freshly ground black
pepper

1/2 cup Chicken Bone Broth
(page 96) or water

Place the onions in the bottom of a 6- to 8-quart slow cooker.

Rinse the pork and pat it dry. Trim off any large pieces of fat.

In a small bowl, combine the garlic, chili powder, oregano, cumin, cayenne, salt, and black pepper. Rub the pork with the spice mixture. Place the pork on top of the onions, add the broth, and cover the slow cooker. Cook on low for about 8 hours.

Place the pork on a platter or cutting board and let rest for 10 minutes. Shred the meat with two forks. Pour some juice over the top and serve.

TUNA CAKES

PREP TIME: **10 MIN.** | COOK TIME: **10 MIN.** | YIELD: **2 SERVINGS** | 1 SERVING = 1 FAT

2 (5-ounce) cans albacore tuna
(in water), drained and broken
up with a fork

1/4 cup minced onion

1 large egg, lightly beaten

2 tablespoons finely chopped
fresh cilantro

1/2 jalapeño, finely chopped
(optional)

2 teaspoons Dijon mustard

1/2 to 1 teaspoon hot sauce

1/4 cup almond flour

1/2 teaspoon Celtic or pink
Himalayan salt (optional; if the
tuna is salted, omit the salt)

Freshly ground black pepper

2 tablespoons avocado oil or
coconut oil

In a medium bowl, combine all the ingredients except the oil, then form the mixture into 8 patties.

In a large skillet, heat the oil over medium heat.

Very gently place 4 patties into the skillet and cook for about 5 minutes, until the patties begin to turn golden on the first side. Very carefully flip the patties using an offset spatula. Cook for 4 to 5 minutes more, and place on a paper towel to drain. Repeat with the remaining 4 patties.

NOTE: These are great served on a bed of lettuce and topped with pico de gallo and/or hot sauce.

Veggies

A fabulous protein deserves an equally yummy side of vegetables. Remember to load your plate with these, because they really ramp up your fat burning.

AVOCADO CUCUMBER SALAD

PREP TIME: **10 MIN.** | YIELD: **2 SERVINGS** | 1 SERVING = 1 FAT

- 2 English cucumbers, halved lengthwise and sliced into half-moons
- 2 celery ribs, diced
- 1/2 small sweet onion, thinly sliced
- 1/2 cup chopped fresh cilantro or Italian parsley
- 1/2 avocado

- 1 tablespoon olive or avocado oil
- 2 tablespoons fresh lemon or lime juice
- Dash of cayenne pepper
- 1/2 teaspoon Celtic or pink Himalayan salt
- 1/4 teaspoon freshly ground black pepper

In a medium bowl, combine the cucumbers, celery, onion, and cilantro.

In a separate bowl, smash the avocado and add the oil, lemon juice, cayenne, salt, and black pepper. Blend together with a fork. If you want a thinner dressing, add a teaspoon or 2 of water.

Pour over the salad and toss well. This is best when it is refrigerated for several hours before serving so the flavors can meld.

NOTES: It's up to you if you want to peel the cucumbers. If you prefer, you can make the dressing in a blender or food processor.

CABBAGE AND BRUSSELS SPROUTS WITH LIME AND CILANTRO

PREP TIME: **10 MIN.** | YIELD: **2 SERVINGS** | 1 SERVING = 1 FAT

2 cups shredded green cabbage

2 cups shredded Brussels sprouts

1 red bell pepper, seeded and cut into matchsticks

1 small sweet onion, thinly sliced

1/2 cup chopped fresh cilantro

2 tablespoons fresh lime juice

2 tablespoons olive or avocado oil

1/4 to 1/2 teaspoon ground cumin

1 garlic clove, minced

1/4 to 1/2 teaspoon hot sauce

1/2 teaspoon Celtic or pink Himalayan salt

1/4 teaspoon freshly ground black pepper

Dash of cayenne pepper

Stevia or monk fruit sweetener, to equal 1 teaspoon sugar

In a large bowl, mix together the cabbage, Brussels sprouts, bell pepper, onion, and cilantro.

In another bowl or a jar with a tight-fitting lid, combine the lime juice, oil, cumin, garlic, hot sauce, salt, black pepper, cayenne, and stevia and whisk/shake well. Pour over the salad and refrigerate. This is best when refrigerated for several hours before serving so the flavors can meld.

NOTE: To save time, you can buy preshredded cabbage and Brussels sprouts. You can also use shredded broccoli as an alternative.

CUCUMBER MINT SALAD

PREP TIME: **10 MIN.** | YIELD: **2 SERVINGS** | 1 SERVING = 1 FAT

2 English cucumbers, halved lengthwise and very thinly sliced into half-moons

1/2 small red onion, very thinly sliced

1/4 cup chopped fresh mint

2 tablespoons olive or avocado oil

2 tablespoons white wine vinegar or champagne vinegar

Stevia or monk fruit sweetener, to equal 2 teaspoons sugar

Dash of cayenne pepper

1/2 teaspoon Celtic or pink Himalayan salt

1/4 teaspoon freshly ground black pepper

Combine the cucumbers, onion, and mint in a medium bowl.

In another bowl or a jar with a tight-fitting lid, combine the oil, vinegar, stevia, cayenne, salt, and black pepper and whisk/shake well. Pour over the salad and toss well. This is best when it is refrigerated for several hours before serving so the flavors can meld.

NOTES: It's up to you if you want to peel the cucumbers.

This Cucumber Mint Salad is also delicious with Sweet Vidalia Onion Vinaigrette (page 119). Just combine the cucumbers, onion, and mint as directed and use the Vidalia vinaigrette in place of the dressing above.

HERB-ROASTED VEGETABLES

PREP TIME: **20 MIN.** | COOK: **45 TO 60 MIN.** | YIELD: **4 SERVINGS** | 1 SERVING = 1 FAT

1 medium onion, thinly sliced

2 zucchini or summer squash, cut into 1/2-inch cubes

1 Chinese eggplant, 2 Japanese eggplants, or 1 small Italian eggplant, cut into 1/2-inch cubes

4 plum tomatoes, seeded and cut into 1/2-inch pieces, or 12 to 16 grape tomatoes, cut in half

2 red or yellow bell peppers, seeded and cut into 1/2-inch cubes

1/4 cup olive or avocado oil

2 garlic cloves, minced, or 1 to 2 teaspoons garlic powder

2 teaspoons Italian seasoning

1 teaspoon Celtic or pink Himalayan salt, plus more as needed

1/2 teaspoon freshly ground black pepper, plus more as needed

Preheat the oven to 375°F.

Put the onion, zucchini, eggplant, tomatoes, and bell peppers into a baking pan that's about 3 inches deep. The vegetables should be about 2 inches deep in the pan. Distribute the oil, garlic, Italian seasoning, salt, and black pepper evenly over the vegetables. Gently toss to distribute the oil.

Bake for 45 to 60 minutes, gently tossing the vegetables once during cooking to move the vegetables on the bottom to the top. Taste and adjust the salt and black pepper to your liking.

WHY ADD PROBIOTICS AND PREBIOTICS TO YOUR SLIM PLATE MEALS?

In Chapter 2, I explained why you need to heal your gut in order to shrink your belly. Now I want to talk about two food groups that can help you make your gut glow: *prebiotics* and *probiotics*.

To understand why it's smart to add these foods to your daily SLIM Plate meals, remember that your gut is an ecosystem that's home to trillions of microbes. And right now I'm guessing this ecosystem is taking a lot of big hits.

Let's start with those three (or was it four?) strawberry daiquiris you downed at that wedding reception last weekend—great fun for you but a total nightmare for your gut bugs. Then add in the NSAIDs you washed down the next day to tame that hangover—drugs that whack those microbes right upside the head.[1]

Now factor in the dose of antibiotics you took for a bladder infection a few weeks ago. That drug poisoned good gut bugs along with the bad ones, slaughtering a host of them. Even more good bugs bought the farm if you ate chicken or steak raised with antibiotics. Ouch.

Then there's all that day-to-day stress—work deadlines, family problems, traffic, bills. This stress toxifies your microbiome, sending your gut bugs into a swoon.

And let's not even talk about what a diet of pizza, take-out burgers, and chips does to them.

Just think about it for a minute. These poor bugs are trapped in your gut their whole lives, working their tiny little butts off for you. And you're *massacring* them by the millions. Even the ones that manage to survive may be sick and struggling.

But relax—because all the foods you'll eat on the 10-Day Belly Slimdown will make these bugs stand up and cheer. And some of the most powerful foods you can feed them are prebiotics and probiotics.

If you're not familiar with these, think of probiotics as the "seeds" in the garden of your microbiome, and pre-biotics as healthy soil in which they can thrive. Here's a look at each one.

- Probiotics are foods or supplements containing live, beneficial microbes that will settle happily into your ecosystem, helping build a diverse and well-balanced microbiome. Probiotic foods include sauerkraut, kim-chi, and pickles. (Be sure to buy unpasteurized ver-sions; you'll find them in the refrigerated section in your grocery or health food store.)

- Prebiotics are foods or supplements high in the solu-ble fiber that your gut microbes love to eat. Prebiotic foods you can eat on this diet include onions, garlic, asparagus, and leeks. (There are starchier ones, such as bananas, jicama, and Jerusalem artichokes, that you can add after you finish your diet.)

SPICY COLESLAW

PREP TIME: **15 MIN.** | YIELD: **2 TO 4 SERVINGS**

4 cups shredded cabbage (green, red, napa, savoy, or any combination)

1 red or yellow bell pepper, seeded and cut into matchsticks

DRESSING

2 tablespoons canned full-fat coconut milk

1 tablespoon coconut aminos

1 1/2 teaspoons unseasoned rice vinegar

1/2 teaspoon grated or minced fresh ginger

3 or 4 scallions, cut into 1/2-inch pieces

1/4 to 1/2 cup roughly chopped fresh Italian parsley or cilantro

2 to 3 teaspoons minced jalapeño or other hot chile pepper

1/8 teaspoon toasted sesame oil (optional)

1/8 teaspoon cayenne pepper

Celtic or pink Himalayan salt

Freshly ground black pepper

Combine the cabbage, bell pepper, scallions, parsley, and jalapeño in a medium bowl.

In another bowl or a jar with a tight-fitting lid, combine the dressing ingredients and whisk/shake well. Season to taste. Pour over the salad and toss. This is best when it is refrigerated for several hours before serving so the flavors can meld.

ASPARAGUS AND TOMATO SALAD

PREP TIME: **10 MIN.** | YIELD: **2 SERVINGS** | 1 SERVING = 1 FAT

1 large bunch asparagus

2 large tomatoes, chopped

1/2 small red onion, thinly sliced

1/4 to 1/2 cup roughly chopped fresh basil

2 tablespoons olive or avocado oil

1 tablespoon red wine vinegar

Celtic or pink Himalayan salt

Freshly ground black pepper

Dash of cayenne pepper

Blanch the asparagus in a pot of simmering water and immediately plunge it into a bowl of ice water. When cool, cut into 1/2- to 1-inch pieces and place in a large bowl.

Add the tomatoes, onion, and basil. Dress with the oil, vinegar, and seasonings. Toss and refrigerate so the flavors can meld.

TOMATO BASIL STACKS

PREP TIME: **5 MIN.** | YIELD: **1 SERVING** | 1 SERVING = 1 FAT

1 large ripe beefsteak tomato, or 2 medium tomatoes, at room temperature

Celtic or pink Himalayan salt

Freshly ground black pepper

8 to 10 fresh basil leaves, julienned

1 tablespoon good-quality olive oil

1 teaspoon balsamic vinegar, or more to taste

Crushed red pepper, for serving (optional)

Slice the tomato horizontally into 1/4-inch-thick slices. Season with salt and black pepper.

Make 1 or more stacks of tomatoes, putting basil between each layer. Drizzle with the olive oil and balsamic vinegar. Add a dash of crushed red pepper, if desired.

VARIATIONS

Add layers of cucumber by slicing lengthwise and cutting to fit the diameter of the tomato slices.

Add layers of thinly sliced sweet onions. Try Vidalia onions when they are in season; they're great!

Serve on a bed of lettuce.

For a nice peppery flavor, serve with arugula or watercress.

Add a handful of roughly chopped fresh parsley.

Instead of olive oil and balsamic vinegar, try Caesar Dressing (page 151).

ZOODLES (ZUCCHINI PASTA) AND MUSHROOMS IN MARINARA SAUCE

PREP TIME: **20 MIN.** | COOK TIME: **10 MIN.** | YIELD: **2 SERVINGS** | 1 SERVING = 1/2 FAT SERVING

1 tablespoon pastured butter or ghee (page 147)

1 1/2 to 2 cups sliced cremini or white mushrooms

2 garlic cloves, minced

2 cups marinara sauce, sugar-free store-bought or homemade (recipe follows)

2 teaspoons dried Italian seasoning, or 2 tablespoons roughly chopped fresh basil, oregano, and/or thyme

1 teaspoon Celtic or pink Himalayan salt

1/2 teaspoon freshly ground black pepper

3 to 4 cups zoodles (from 3 to 4 small to medium zucchini; see Note, page 109), at room temperature

Crushed red pepper, for serving (optional)

Fresh basil, julienned, for serving (optional)

In a large skillet or Dutch oven, melt the butter over medium heat. Add the mushrooms and cook, stirring, for about 5 minutes, until the mushrooms soften. After 3 minutes, add the garlic so it softens but doesn't brown.

Add the marinara sauce, herbs, salt, and black pepper and bring to a simmer. Taste and adjust the seasoning to your taste. Pour the sauce over the zoodles and serve with crushed red pepper and basil, if desired.

NOTE: Zoodles can get mushy very quickly. If the zucchini is at room temperature, the heat of the sauce alone will warm the zoodles sufficiently. You can stir the zoodles into the sauce and serve immediately. If you refrigerate leftovers with the zoodles in the sauce, water from the zucchini will thin the sauce.

VARIATION

If you want to turn this into a One-Pot Bolognese Meal, add 1/2 pound ground beef, ground turkey, or sugar-, nitrate- and nitrite-free sausage. Use avocado oil instead of butter and brown the meat first and set aside. Add it to the pan when you add the marinara sauce.

HOW TO MAKE GHEE

A number of these recipes call for *ghee,* also called *clarified butter.* You can buy ghee in many health food stores—one of my favorite brands is Eat Good Fat ghee—but it's also a cinch to make it at home. Simply heat a stick of butter gently, then skim off the milk solids with a mesh strainer when they come to the top. Cool the ghee and keep it refrigerated.

QUICK-AND-EASY MARINARA SAUCE

1 (15-ounce) can diced tomatoes

1/2 cup tomato sauce (half an 8-ounce can tomato sauce)

1 or 2 garlic cloves, minced

2 tablespoons roughy chopped fresh Italian parsley, or more to taste

1 teaspoon dried Italian seasoning, or 1 tablespoon roughly chopped fresh basil, oregano, and/or thyme, or more to taste

1/2 teaspoon Celtic or pink Himalayan salt

1/4 teaspoon freshly ground black pepper, plus more to taste

Crushed red pepper

Combine all the ingredients in a saucepan and simmer on low for 20 minutes.

Putting It All Together:
A Perfect Plate

These recipes contain the protein, veggies, and fat for your evening meal. Add a handful of berries or half a grapefruit, and you're ready to eat!

CHIPOTLE CHICKEN WRAPS

PREP TIME: **3 MIN.** | YIELD: **1 SERVING** | 1 SERVING = 1 FAT

1 tablespoon avocado oil mayonnaise

1 teaspoon canned chipotle chiles in adobo sauce (be sure to use some of the sauce), or more to taste

Squeeze of fresh lime

3 or 4 romaine leaves or other large-leaf lettuce

1 cooked chicken breast, or 4 to 6 ounces chicken from a rotisserie chicken or Roast Chicken with Herbs and Lemon (page 135), sliced or shredded

Salt and freshly ground black pepper

OPTIONAL TOPPINGS

Sliced tomato

Sliced onions

Chopped cilantro

Sliced red and yellow bell peppers

Sliced scallions

Hot sauce

Combine the mayonnaise, chipotles in adobo, and lime juice in a small bowl.

Place the lettuce leaves on a flat surface and top with the sauce, chicken, and any of the toppings you like. Season with salt and pepper and roll up or fold in half.

AVOCADO TUNA SALAD

PREP TIME: **5 MIN.** | YIELD: **1 SERVING** | 1 SERVING = 1 FAT

1/4 to 1/2 avocado

1 celery rib, diced

2 tablespoons diced red onion

1 teaspoon Dijon mustard

2 teaspoons fresh lemon or lime juice, plus more if needed

1/2 teaspoon dried dill

1/8 teaspoon ground cumin

Dash of cayenne pepper

1 (5-ounce) can albacore tuna (in water), drained and broken up with a fork

Celtic or pink Himalayan salt (optional)

Freshly ground black pepper (optional)

Smash the avocado in a medium bowl and add the celery, onion, mustard, lemon juice, dill, cumin, and cayenne. Blend with a fork. Add the tuna and mix together. If you want a thinner dressing, add water or lemon juice by the teaspoon until you get the desired consistency. Taste and add salt and black pepper, if desired.

SERVING IDEAS: Enjoy on a bed of lettuce, stuffed in a tomato, or served with crudités.

CHICKEN WITH CREAMY CILANTRO SAUCE

PREP TIME: **10 MIN.** | YIELD: **2 SERVINGS** | 1 SERVING = 1 FAT

1/2 avocado

1 tablespoon avocado oil mayonnaise

1/4 to 1/3 cup packed fresh cilantro leaves, roughly chopped

1 tablespoon fresh lime juice

1 small garlic clove, minced

Dash of cayenne pepper

Celtic or pink Himalayan salt

Freshly ground black pepper

8 ounces cooked chicken from a rotisserie chicken or Roast Chicken with Herbs and Lemon (page 135), diced or shredded

2 celery ribs, diced

2 tablespoons minced yellow onion

4 to 6 cups lettuce, your choice, or 1 head large-leaf lettuce such as Bibb if you choose to make wraps

8 or more radishes, thinly sliced

Place the avocado, mayonnaise, cilantro, lime juice, garlic, and cayenne in a blender or food processor and blend until smooth and creamy. If you want a thinner dressing, add a teaspoon or more of water or lime juice until desired consistency is reached. Taste and season with salt and black pepper.

Combine the chicken, celery, and onion in a small bowl. Toss with the dressing. Serve over lettuce or as lettuce wraps with sliced radishes.

VARIATION

Blend 2 to 3 teaspoons canned chipotles in adobo or smoked paprika into the cilantro sauce for a smoky hit of spice! Chipotles in adobo is sold in small cans found in the Hispanic food section of most grocers.

BUTTER LETTUCE WITH AVOCADO EGG SALAD

PREP TIME: **10 MIN.** | YIELD: **1 SERVING** | 1 SERVING = 1 FAT

2 or 3 hard-boiled eggs, diced

1/4 avocado

1 1/2 teaspoons avocado oil mayonnaise

1 teaspoon Dijon mustard

Dash of cayenne pepper or hot sauce

Fresh lemon juice (optional)

4 to 6 leaves butter lettuce (or your favorite lettuce)

1 medium tomato, diced

Celtic or pink Himalayan salt (optional)

Freshly ground black pepper (optional)

Combine the eggs, avocado, mayonnaise, Dijon, and cayenne in a small bowl. If you want the egg salad thinner, add a teaspoon or 2 of water or lemon juice.

Pile the egg salad evenly on the lettuce leaves and top with the tomatoes. Add salt and black pepper, if desired. Roll up or fold in half.

SERVING SUGGESTION: Enjoy with a variety of crunchy raw vegetables.

CHICKEN CAESAR SALAD

PREP TIME: **10 MIN.** | YIELD: **2 SERVINGS** | 1 ROUNDED TABLESPOON DRESSING = 1 FAT SERVING

CAESAR DRESSING

2 garlic cloves, finely minced

1/2 teaspoon Dijon mustard

1 tablespoon fresh lemon juice

1 tablespoon avocado oil mayonnaise

1 teaspoon Worcestershire sauce or coconut aminos

1 teaspoon anchovy paste

1/4 cup olive oil

1/2 to 1 teaspoon capers (optional)

Celtic or pink Himalayan salt

Freshly ground black pepper

SALAD

1 large, or 2 small heads romaine lettuce, cut or torn

8 ounces cooked chicken, shredded or cut into strips

Make the dressing: Combine the garlic, mustard, lemon juice, mayonnaise, Worcestershire, and anchovy paste in a medium bowl and blend into a creamy paste. Very slowly whisk in the oil until all the ingredients are fully incorporated. Add the capers, if using. Taste and add salt and pepper.

Put the lettuce in a large bowl. Add a rounded tablespoon of the Caesar dressing and toss with tongs to coat the lettuce. Portion evenly on two plates, top with the chicken, and serve with pepper.

Refrigerate the remaining dressing. It will stay fresh for at least 1 week.

VARIATION

To make a Chipotle Caesar Dressing, replace the anchovy paste with 2 to 3 teaspoons canned chipotles in adobo and a dash of hot sauce or cayenne, and replace the lemon juice with lime juice. Add the chipotles in adobo when you make the creamy paste in the first step of this recipe.

NOTES: The dressing makes 4 to 5 servings. Store in a sealed container in the refrigerator for up to 1 week. Feel free to add any other vegetables on the approved list to your salad if you choose. It's really good with roasted red peppers!

COBB SALAD

PREP TIME: **5 MIN.** | YIELD: **1 SERVING** | 1 SERVING = 1 FAT

2 to 3 cups cut or torn lettuce (any type)

2 to 3 ounces cooked chicken from a rotisserie chicken or Roast Chicken with Herbs and Lemon (page 135), or 2 to 3 ounces roast turkey or sugar-, nitrate-, and nitrite-free deli turkey breast

1 medium tomato, diced

$1/2$ cucumber, diced

1 hard-boiled egg, diced

$1/4$ to $1/2$ avocado, cubed

Juice of $1/2$ lemon (about 2 tablespoons)

Celtic or pink Himalayan salt

Freshly ground black pepper

Place all the ingredients in a medium bowl and toss. The egg yolk combined with avocado and lemon juice will create a creamy, flavorful dressing. Season with salt and pepper to taste.

NOTE: Although Cobb salads are usually composed, tossing it all together creates the dressing for this salad. Easy!

SPICY EGG SALAD

PREP TIME: **10 MIN.** | YIELD: **1 SERVING** | 1 FAT SERVING = 1 FAT

2 to 3 hard-boiled eggs, diced

1 tablespoon avocado oil mayonnaise

2 tablespoons pico de gallo, or more to taste

2 to 4 tablespoons roughly chopped fresh cilantro

Squeeze of fresh lime juice

$1/4$ teaspoon chili powder

Dash of hot sauce or cayenne pepper

Celtic or pink Himalayan salt

Freshly ground black pepper

Combine the eggs, mayonnaise, pico de gallo, cilantro, lime juice, chili powder, and hot sauce in a small bowl and mix with a fork. If you want the egg salad spicier, add more hot sauce. If you like it chunkier, add more pico de gallo. Taste and season with salt and black pepper.

SERVING SUGGESTION: Enjoy with a variety of crunchy raw vegetables, on top of a salad, or in lettuce wraps.

TURKEY WRAPS WITH GREEN GODDESS DRESSING

PREP TIME: **10 MIN.** | YIELD: **2 SERVINGS** | 1 SERVING = 1 FAT

GREEN GODDESS DRESSING

$1/2$ avocado

1 tablespoon avocado oil mayonnaise

1 tablespoon chopped fresh chives

2 to 3 teaspoons chopped fresh tarragon

1 teaspoon anchovy paste

$1^1/2$ teaspoons fresh lemon juice, plus more if needed

Celtic or pink Himalayan salt

Freshly ground black pepper

WRAPS

8 ounces or more sliced turkey breast or sugar-, nitrite-, and nitrate-free deli turkey breast

4 to 8 large lettuce leaves

2 medium tomatoes, diced

1 cucumber, peeled, seeded, and diced

Make the dressing: Place the avocado, mayo, chives, tarragon, anchovy paste, and lemon juice in a blender or food processor and blend until smooth and creamy. If you want a thinner dressing, add a teaspoon or more of water or lemon juice until the desired consistency is reached. Taste and season with salt and pepper.

Place a slice of turkey atop each lettuce leaf, spread with Green Goddess dressing, top with diced tomatoes and cucumber, and roll up to create a turkey wrap.

NOTES: Green Goddess dressing is also fabulous on a garden salad, served with fish or chicken, or used as a crudité dip.

In a hurry? You can use 1 tablespoon avocado mayonnaise instead of the Green Goddess dressing, or you could skip the mayo and use $1/4$ to $1/2$ avocado per person.

One-Pot Meals

Love meals that come together in a single pot or pan, making meal prep and cleanup a breeze? Then I've got your number here!

CHICKEN TERIYAKI WITH VEGETABLES

PREP TIME: **20 MIN.** | COOK TIME: **15 MIN.** | YIELD: **4 SERVINGS** | 1 SERVING = 1 FAT

Technically, this is a two-pot meal, because you'll need a little saucepan at first. But you'll forgive my tiny cheat when you discover how delicious this is!

TERIYAKI SAUCE

1/2 cup coconut aminos

2 tablespoons unseasoned rice vinegar

1 (1-inch) knob fresh ginger, peeled and grated

1 garlic clove, minced

Stevia or monk fruit sweetener to equal 11/2 to 2 tablespoons sugar

1/2 to 1 teaspoon arrowroot powder

1/8 teaspoon crushed red pepper

CHICKEN AND VEGETABLES

4 tablespoons coconut oil or avocado oil

11/4 pounds boneless, skinless chicken breasts or thighs, cut into 1-inch cubes

2 cups broccoli florets

2 cups thinly sliced baby bok choy (about 5)

2 cups thinly sliced savoy or napa cabbage (about 1/2 head)

1 red bell pepper, seeded and cut into strips

1 cup sliced mushrooms (see Notes)

3 scallions, cut into 1/2-inch pieces

1/4 cup roughly chopped fresh cilantro (optional)

Make the teriyaki sauce. Combine all the ingredients and 1/4 cup water in a small saucepan and heat over medium heat, stirring occasionally, until the mixture thickens. Taste and the adjust the sweetness to your liking. Cover to keep warm and set aside.

Make the chicken and vegetables. Heat 1 tablespoon of the oil in a wok or large skillet over medium-high to high heat. Add the chicken and quickly stir-fry so all sides are browned, 3 to 4 minutes. Remove from the pan and set aside.

Add another tablespoon of oil to the pan and stir-fry the broccoli for about 3 minutes so it is cooked but still very crisp. Remove from the pan and set aside with the chicken.

Add another tablespoon of oil to the pan and stir-fry the bok choy and cabbage. Remove from the pan and set aside with the chicken and broccoli.

Add the remaining 1 tablespoon oil to the pan and stir-fry the bell pepper, mushrooms, and scallions.

Combine all the ingredients in a serving bowl, pour the teriyaki sauce over the chicken and vegetables, and toss to coat. Top with the cilantro, if using.

NOTES: To save time you can buy precut stir-fry vegetables. You can also use any combination of vegetables from the approved vegetables list (page 47). If you cook the vegetables in batches, you can keep the vegetables crisp. If you put all the vegetables in the pan at once, they will steam, not fry.

Teriyaki sauce can be used in many ways. Brush it on salmon, chicken, beef, or pork before sautéing, baking, or broiling. Pour it over steamed vegetables for extra flavor. Use it over vegetables and cauliflower "rice" for a tasty rice bowl.

Instead of the vegetables used in this recipe, use 8 cups of your choice of Asian stir-fry vegetables, available already precut and packed at many grocers.

CHICKEN WITH BRUSSELS SPROUTS

PREP TIME: **20 MIN.** | COOK TIME: **30 MIN.** | YIELD: **4 SERVINGS** | 1 SERVING = 1 FAT

4 boneless, skinless chicken thighs or breasts

1/4 to 1/2 teaspoon ground sage

1/2 teaspoon smoked paprika (optional, if you like a smoky flavor)

Celtic or pink Himalayan salt

Freshly ground black pepper

1 tablespoon coconut oil or avocado oil

6 cups Brussels sprouts, cut in quarters or halves, or 6 cups small cauliflower and broccoli florets

1 shallot, thinly sliced

1/3 cup Chicken Bone Broth (page 96)

Preheat the oven to 400°F and place a rack in the middle of the oven.

Season the chicken with the sage, paprika (if using), and salt and pepper to taste. In an oven-safe skillet, heat the oil. Add the chicken and cook for 4 to 5 minutes per side for breasts or 3 to 4 minutes for thighs, turning only once. Remove the chicken and set aside.

Add the vegetables and shallot to the pan and toss well. Cook for 3 to 4 minutes, until they start to soften. Return the chicken to the pan on top of the vegetables, add the broth, cover, and place in the oven.

Bake for 10 to 15 minutes, until the chicken is fully cooked and no longer pink inside (165°F). Remove from the oven and serve.

NOTE: You can cook this recipe entirely on the stovetop on low heat, but you may need to add a bit more broth.

FRITTATA WITH HAM, LEEKS, ASPARAGUS, AND MUSHROOMS

PREP TIME: **20 MIN.** | COOK TIME: **20 TO 25 MIN.** | YIELD: **4 SERVINGS** | 1 SERVING = 1/2 FAT SERVING

2 tablespoons ghee (page 147), coconut oil, or avocado oil

2 leeks, white and pale green parts only, thinly sliced

1 pound or more asparagus, trimmed and cut into 1-inch pieces

8 ounces mushrooms, thinly sliced

8 large eggs

1 teaspoon dried thyme, or use any of your favorite herbs

Dash of ground nutmeg (optional)

1/2 to 1 teaspoon Celtic or pink Himalayan salt

1/2 teaspoon freshly ground black pepper

1/2 pound ham, cut into cubes, or fully cooked nitrate-, nitrite-, and sugar-free sausage, cut into 1/2-inch rounds

Preheat the oven to 350°F and position a rack in the top third of the oven.

In a 10- to 12-inch cast-iron skillet or other oven-safe skillet, heat 1 tablespoon of the ghee over medium heat. Add the leeks and cook for about 5 minutes, stirring occasionally, until softened. Add the asparagus and cook for about 5 more minutes. Add the remaining 1 tablespoon ghee and the mushrooms and raise the heat to medium-high. Cook until any liquid has evaporated from the pan, 5 to 6 minutes.

While the vegetables are cooking, whisk together the eggs, thyme, nutmeg, salt, and pepper. Add the ham to the pan of vegetables and pour the eggs evenly over the entire pan. Stir to evenly distribute the meat and vegetables. Cook for about 5 minutes, until the eggs begin to set around the edges.

Remove the pan from the stovetop and place in the oven. Bake for 20 to 25 minutes, until the frittata is golden brown. To test for doneness, insert a knife into the center of the frittata. If the eggs are runny, return to the oven and check again every 5 minutes.

NOTES: Any vegetables will do; just be sure they are precooked to release their water so your frittata isn't soggy. It's also a great way to use up leftover meat or vegetables you may have in the refrigerator. If you prepared the pork in the batch-cooking section, you can use that instead of ham.

LEMON ROSEMARY CHICKEN WITH CAULIFLOWER "RICE"

PREP TIME: **15 MIN.** | COOK TIME: **30 MIN.** | YIELD: **4 SERVINGS** | 1 SERVING = 1/2 FAT SERVING

6 boneless, skinless chicken thighs

Zest of 2 lemons

Juice of 1/2 lemon

2 tablespoons chopped fresh rosemary leaves, or 2 teaspoons dried rosemary

2 garlic cloves, minced

1 teaspoon Celtic or pink Himalayan salt

1/2 teaspoon freshly ground black pepper

2 tablespoons coconut oil or avocado oil

1 cup Chicken Bone Broth (page 96)

4 to 6 cups cauliflower "rice" (see Note)

1/4 cup roughly chopped fresh Italian parsley

Combine the chicken, half the lemon zest, the lemon juice, half the rosemary, the garlic, salt, and pepper in a medium nonaluminum bowl or a large food storage bag. Refrigerate to marinate for 30 minutes to 1 hour.

In a small bowl, combine the parsley and the remaining lemon zest and rosemary. Set aside.

Heat the oil in a large skillet or Dutch oven over medium-high heat. Add the chicken and cook for about 4 minutes per side, turning only once. Add 1/2 cup of the broth, cover, and reduce the heat to medium. Simmer for about 10 minutes.

Remove the chicken from the pan, add the cauliflower "rice," and stir to coat. Top with the remaining 1/2 cup broth, and put the chicken on top of the cauliflower.

Cover and simmer on medium to medium-low heat for about 15 minutes, until the chicken is fully cooked and the cauliflower is tender. To serve, sprinkle the reserved lemon-herb mixture over the chicken. Serve with lemon wedges, if desired.

NOTE: Riced cauliflower is a fabulous substitute for brown or white rice and very quick and easy to make. Simply remove florets from the stem, place in a food processor, and pulse until it looks like rice. You may need to do two batches if it is a large cauliflower. Many grocers now sell cauliflower "rice" bagged in the produce section.

NO-BEAN CHILI

PREP TIME: **20 MIN.** | COOK TIME: **30 MIN.** | YIELD: **4 SERVINGS** | 1 SERVING = 1/2 FAT SERVING

2 tablespoons avocado oil

1 1/4 pounds lean ground beef or ground sirloin

1 medium sweet onion, diced

1 celery rib, diced

2 garlic cloves, minced, or 1 teaspoon garlic powder

2 cups diced zucchini (about 4 small)

1 to 2 tablespoons chili powder

1 teaspoon ground cumin

1/2 teaspoon dried oregano (optional)

Dash of ground cinnamon (optional)

1 teaspoon Celtic or pink Himalayan salt

1/2 teaspoon freshly ground black pepper

1/4 teaspoon cayenne pepper

1 (28-ounce) can diced tomatoes

1/2 cup Beef (page 95) or Chicken (page 96) Bone Broth

1/2 cup roughly chopped fresh cilantro

Heat the oil in a large skillet or Dutch oven over medium-high heat. When the oil is hot, add the beef and cook, stirring, until cooked through. Add the onion, celery, and garlic to the pan. Cook for 3 to 4 minutes, until they begin to soften. Add the zucchini, chili powder, cumin, oregano, cinnamon, salt, black pepper, cayenne, tomatoes, and broth. Stir to combine.

Bring to a boil, immediately reduce the heat to low, and simmer for about 20 minutes. Stir in the cilantro just before serving.

SERVING SUGGESTIONS: This chili is great served over cauliflower "rice" (see Note, page 158).

For great toppings, try diced sweet onions or chopped scallions, cubed avocado, or sliced pitted California black olives.

VARIATIONS

If you prefer a chunkier chili, you can substitute brisket for the ground beef. Just trim the fat and cut the meat into ½-inch cubes. You can also substitute ground turkey or a combination of ground beef and ground pork.

You can also make a No-Bean White Chili with a few small changes to this recipe: Use ground turkey or chicken instead of beef. Substitute 1 to 2 diced poblano peppers for the celery. Omit the canned tomatoes and use 2 (4-ounce) cans diced green chiles with liquid. Add 2 cups Chicken Bone Broth (page 96).

NEW TO STEAMING VEGGIES? HERE'S HOW TO DO IT.

I come from a big Italian family, and I started cooking as soon as I could stand on a chair on tiptoe to reach the stovetop. I'm no Giada De Laurentiis, but I can do an Italian wedding soup that's *molto delizioso* and a pesto that's to die for.

However, some of my closest friends (especially those in the Big Apple) don't set foot in the kitchen except to hit "start" on the cappuccino machine. Open their fridges and you'll find sparkling water, a half-empty bottle of Chardonnay, and a whole lot of takeout boxes. Basically, their idea of "cooking" is to phone for moo goo gai pan and unwrap the chopsticks before they eat it.

If you're like these buds of mine, I know that the idea of cooking lots of veggies every day might alarm you. If so, I have good news: Cooking non-starchy vegetables is *easy*! You don't need any fancy equipment, and you don't need mad kitchen skills. In fact, if you can turn on a stove burner or an oven, you're already overqualified for the job.

Here are two ways—both simple and stress-free—to steam those veggies in just minutes.

STEAMING ON THE STOVE

Wash and prep your veggies. Place a steamer or a metal colander inside a pot with a cover. Add about an inch of water, making sure the steamer or colander is above the water level, and cover the pan. When the water boils, add your vegetables to the pan, pop on the lid, and reduce the heat.

Different veggies cook at different rates—for instance, asparagus takes longer than spinach—so check occasionally and see how your vegetables are coming along. You want them to be bright and vibrant and still have some "crunch."

When your veggies are done, put them on a plate or sheet pan in a single layer to cool. They'll keep cooking for a few minutes; if you want them to stop cooking right away, toss them into an ice water bath for a few seconds. Sprinkle on a little sea salt or Himalayan pink salt, and you're ready to go.

STEAMING IN THE OVEN

Start by preheating your oven to 350°F, and put the vegetables in a roasting pan or Dutch oven with about a half inch of water or preferably bone broth. (This bone broth will be a treasure trove of nutrients when you're done cooking, so save it and drink it.)

Cover your pan tightly with foil or with the lid to the pan. Cook for 5 minutes, and then take a peek at your veggies every few minutes. When they're done, place them on a plate or sheet pan in a single layer to cool if you don't plan to eat them immediately. (They'll keep cooking for a few minutes after you take them from the oven.) A dash of sea salt or pink Himalayan salt will finish them perfectly.

TIPS

- It may take one or two tries to get your veggies exactly right. However, if you overcook leafy veggies a little and they get "mushy," they'll still work great in your afternoon broth—so don't throw them out!

- If you want to steam several vegetables at the same time, pick veggies that play well together. For instance, broccoli and cauliflower are a great pair because they cook in the same amount of time, but zucchini and broccoli aren't a good match because the zucchini cooks much faster than the broccoli.

PORK WITH CRUNCHY ASIAN VEGETABLES

PREP TIME: **20 MIN.** | COOK TIME: **10 MIN.** | YIELD: **2 SERVINGS** | 1 SERVING = 1 FAT

2 tablespoons coconut oil or avocado oil

1/2 pound Slow Cooker Pulled Pork (page 138), or 1/2 pound pork tenderloin, cut into 1-inch cubes

1 garlic clove, minced, or 1/4 to 1/2 teaspoon garlic powder

2 cups 1-inch pieces bok choy

2 cups broccoli florets

1 cup snow peas

2 or 3 scallions, cut into 1/2-inch pieces

2 tablespoons coconut aminos

1/2 cup roughly chopped fresh cilantro

Freshly ground black or white pepper

1 or 2 teaspoons arrowroot powder (optional)

1/2 cup Beef (page 95) or Chicken (page 96) Bone Broth or water (optional)

Heat the oil in a large skillet over medium-high heat. Add the pork cubes and garlic and brown for 4 to 5 minutes on all sides. (If you are using Slow Cooker Pulled Pork, you will add it at the end.)

Raise the heat to high and add the bok choy and broccoli. Cook, stirring, for about 3 minutes. Add the snow peas, scallions, and coconut aminos and cook for 2 to 3 minutes; you want the vegetables to still have some crunch. Add the cilantro and pepper to taste and serve with additional coconut aminos.

If you are using the pork loin you already cooked, add as the last step and gently stir to coat the meat.

To thicken the sauce, mix the arrowroot into the broth or water, add to the pan, and bring to a simmer. Simmer until the sauce thickens.

VARIATIONS

You can use any of your favorite vegetables from the approved vegetables list on page 47 in addition to or instead of those noted here.

Optionally, add about 1/2 teaspoon Chinese five-spice powder for additional seasoning.

You can also serve over cauliflower "rice" (see Note, page 158) or zoodles if you choose.

If you like it spicy, add 1 tablespoon minced seeded jalapeño or use crushed red pepper or sriracha when serving.

SKILLET CHICKEN, CHILI, AND LIME

PREP TIME: **20 MIN.** | COOK TIME: **30 TO 35 MIN.** | YIELD: **4 SERVINGS** | 1 SERVING = 1/2 FAT SERVING

1 tablespoon chili powder

1 teaspoon ground cumin

2 garlic cloves, minced, or 1 teaspoon garlic powder

1/4 teaspoon cayenne pepper

Dash of ground cinnamon

1 teaspoon Celtic or pink Himalayan salt

1/2 teaspoon freshly ground black pepper

6 boneless, skinless chicken thighs

2 tablespoons avocado oil or coconut oil

1 cup Chicken Bone Broth (page 96)

4 to 6 cups cauliflower "rice" (see Note, page 158)

2 limes, 1 juiced and 1 cut into wedges for serving

1/4 cup roughly chopped fresh cilantro

In a small bowl, combine the chili powder, cumin, garlic, cayenne, cinnamon, salt, and black pepper. Rub the chicken with this mixture, coating all sides.

In a large skillet or Dutch oven, heat the oil over medium-high heat. Add the chicken, reduce the heat to medium, and cook for about 4 minutes per side, turning once. Monitor the heat, as the spices will burn if it's too high. Add 1/2 cup of the broth, cover, and reduce the heat to medium-low. Simmer for about 15 minutes.

Remove the chicken from the pan, add the cauliflower "rice" and any remaining spice mix, and stir in the remaining ½ cup broth. Place the chicken on top of the cauliflower. Cover and simmer on medium-low heat for about 15 minutes, until the chicken is fully cooked.

When done, drizzle the lime juice over the chicken and top with the cilantro. Serve with the lime wedges.

TUSCAN CHICKEN

PREP TIME: **20 MIN.** | COOK TIME: **30 MIN.** | YIELD: **4 SERVINGS** | 1 SERVING = 1/2 FAT SERVING

1 tablespoon coconut oil or avocado oil

4 to 6 boneless, skinless chicken thighs (1¼ to 1½ pounds), cut into 1-inch cubes

½ medium onion, sliced

4 red and/or yellow bell peppers, seeded and cut into 1-inch pieces

2 garlic cloves, minced

1 teaspoon Italian seasoning

1 (24-ounce) jar sugar-free marinara sauce or homemade marinara (page 147)

16 pitted California black olives, halved

Celtic or pink Himalayan salt

Freshly ground black pepper

4 cups zoodles (about 4 small to medium zucchini; see Note, page 146), at room temperature

Fresh basil, julienned, for serving (optional)

Crushed red pepper, for serving (optional)

In a large skillet or Dutch oven, heat the oil over medium-high heat. Add the chicken and cook for 3 to 4 minutes per side, turning only once. Transfer the chicken to a plate and set aside.

Return the pan to the heat, add the onion and bell peppers, and sauté for about 5 minutes, until the vegetables just begin to soften. Add the garlic and Italian seasoning and cook for 5 minutes. Pour in the marinara and add the chicken. Reduce the heat to low, cover, and simmer for about 10 minutes. Stir in the olives and simmer for 10 minutes more. Taste the sauce and add salt and black pepper to taste. Serve over the zoodles, topped with fresh basil and crushed red pepper, if desired.

NOTES: Zoodles can get mushy very quickly when cooking. If the zoodles are at room temperature, the heat of the sauce alone will warm them. You can stir the zoodles into the sauce, but if you have leftovers, water from the zucchini will thin the sauce.

You can also serve this dish with cauliflower "rice" (see Note, page 158).

UNSTUFFED CABBAGE

PREP TIME: **15 MIN.** | COOK TIME: **35 MIN.** | YIELD: **4 SERVINGS**

1 tablespoon coconut oil or avocado oil

1 1/4 pounds ground beef or ground sirloin

1 medium onion, diced

1 garlic clove, minced

8 to 9 cups roughly chopped cabbage (about 1 medium head)

1 (28-ounce) can diced tomatoes

1 cup Chicken (page 96) or Beef (page 95) Bone Broth

1 teaspoon Hungarian paprika

1 1/2 teaspoons Celtic or pink Himalayan salt

1 teaspoon freshly ground black pepper

In large skillet or Dutch oven, heat the oil over medium-high heat. When the oil is hot, add the beef and cook, stirring often, for 5 to 7 minutes, until browned and cooked through.

Add the remaining ingredients, stir to combine, and reduce the heat to medium-low. Cover and simmer for about 30 minutes, until the cabbage is soft.

VARIATION

After simmering for 15 minutes, add 2 cups cauliflower "rice" (see Note, page 158).

THREE MORE BELLY-BLASTING "POWER-UPS"

My belly-slimming exercises will give you a sculpted waist, my powerful stress-reduction strategies will help you cut your cravings and keep those pounds off forever, and my detox regimen will sweep away the toxins that make your belly fat and old.

SCULPT YOUR ABS WITH TARGETED EXERCISES

On the 10-Day Belly Slimdown, you're going to *blast* your belly fat by increasing your fasting hours and kicking your metabolism into hyperdrive. When you do eat, you're going to melt off even more fat with beautiful bone broth and SLIM-gestion foods.

And guess what: I have even *more* belly-blasting power for you! In this chapter, I'll tell you how exercise can help make your abs sleek and beautiful.

However, here's something I want you to know up front. The 10-Day Belly Slimdown is a tough "boot camp" diet—I totally admit this—and the diet alone is going to give you incredible results whether you exercise or not. That's because the real magic lies in shrinking your eating window.

So during your ten-day diet, I want you to focus your attention on your eating plan. If you feel like exercising, that's great. If not, just do a little gentle walking or stretching. Then, after your diet is over, you can start a more challenging regimen.

Above all, I really don't want you to hit a wall during your diet and begin getting discouraged. On Days 4 through 7 in particular, when you may be experiencing the "carb flu" (see page 71), I want you to take it easy on your body.

Also, remember that exercise takes longer than diet to slim your belly, so be patient. Keep it up, and you'll start to see a big difference within six to twelve weeks.

And here's news that will make you happy: You don't need to spend hours doing crunches to get gorgeous abs. Instead, you can pick and choose from these easy, fun, and effective belly-trimming strategies.

Deep Breathing

I'm betting you already know that deep breathing is a powerful way to relieve your stress. But did you know that it's a fantastic way to fight belly fat, too?

Deep breathing—also called *abdominal breathing* or *primal breathing*—tones and tightens the abs. In particular, it's great for getting rid of that annoying post-pregnancy "pooch" that new moms hate so much.

In addition, when you do deep breathing, you trigger a "relaxation response." This response actually *alters your gene expression* in ways that reduce inflammation, improve your metabolism, and lower your insulin levels.[1] All this, in turn, ramps up fat burning.

Want more benefits? Deep breathing clears your mind, lowers your blood pressure, helps clean toxins out of your system, and strengthens your immune system.

Pretty cool, right? What's more, you can practice deep breathing anytime, anywhere—and it's easy. Here's how to do it.

- Get into a comfortable position.

- Inhale deeply through your nose for the count of five. Be sure to "belly breathe," expanding your belly as much as possible. It may help to visualize your belly inflating like a balloon.

- Pause for two counts and then exhale through your mouth. Rather than forcing the air out, release it slowly to the count of five, pulling your belly button back toward your spine. Pause for two seconds before breathing in again.

- If you like, say a soothing word or syllable each time you breathe out.

- Repeat your deep breaths about ten times, and you'll feel the relaxation response kicking in.

Practice deep breathing several times each day, and over time you'll naturally start breathing more deeply all day long. I'm not exaggerating when I say that this is one of the most important "slim belly forever" habits you can cultivate.

The Stomach Vacuum

Here's another of those "two-fers" I love. In addition to giving your abs a powerful workout while you're doing it, this exercise will train you to keep your tummy tucked in during the day.

To do this exercise, pick a time when you haven't eaten recently. Choose one of these positions:

- On your back, with your knees bent and your feet flat on the floor.

- On your hands and knees.

- Sitting up straight in a chair with no armrests.

Take a few deep breaths. Then exhale as much air as you can, and pull your belly button in toward your spine. Hold this position for 15 seconds, squeezing your belly button in as far as you can and taking small breaths if needed. Try to work your way up to 60 seconds.

Afterward, throughout the day, do mini-versions of this exercise. A dozen or so times each day, pull your belly button toward your spine for a count of five or ten.

Ten Thousand Steps

To get more exercise in an easy way, track how much you're walking with a pedometer or step-tracking app. See if you can walk at least ten thousand steps per day; it's easier than you think. For instance, you can multitask by walking in place while you binge-watch your favorite shows. Every mile you rack up will burn off calories and lower your insulin levels,[2] taking off belly fat.

If you and your partner are both trying to lose weight, consider making a friendly competition out of your daily steps, with the winner getting to hand off a chore such as washing the dishes or taking out the trash. (This is also a fun way to get your kids off the couch and onto their feet.) And to burn even more fat, try walking faster or walking up an incline.

HIIT Training

In a HIIT (high-intensity interval training) workout, you alternate short bursts of intense activity with periods of recovery. HIIT is a strenuous form of exercise, so feel free to save it for after your diet.

HIIT is hugely popular these days because it's great for your cardiovascular system, and new research shows that it's a belly-blaster, as well. For instance:

- A study of postmenopausal women with type 2 diabetes compared the effects of continuous, moderate cycling to HIIT involving bursts of intense cycling followed by recovery periods. Both groups lost fat mass, but the researchers say that "significant loss of total abdominal and visceral fat mass was observed only with HIIT."[3]

- In a second study, this time involving overweight men, researchers in Australia looked at the effects of HIIT workouts performed on an exercise bike. They found that just one hour a week of this activity burned the same amount of body fat as jogging for seven hours a week! Better yet, participants primarily lost visceral fat. While this study only involved men, the researchers said women were getting the same results.[4]

One reason HIIT is so effective is that the intense intervals give your core muscles a real challenge. (Try biking or running in place

---

FOUR WAYS EXERCISE BATTLES BELLY FAT

- *Exercise keeps your metabolism soaring even* after *you finish.* After high-intensity exercise, your body needs to recover. Recovery takes work, and work takes energy. So long after you exercise, your metabolism stays revved up, and you burn extra calories.

- *Exercise turns white fat into brown fat.* Did you know that you want *more* brown fat? Instead of storing calories, brown fat burns them. When you exercise, levels of the hormone irisin and a metabolic regulator called FGF21 rise. These turn white fat cells into brown fat cells, and that in turn ramps up calorie burning.[5]

- *Exercise builds muscle.* Muscle burns more calories than fat does. So the more lean muscle you create through exercise, the more calories you'll burn all day long.

- *Exercise energizes you, so you move more—and move faster.* Exercise fires up your cells, revitalizing you. Without even thinking about it, you'll get even more active and burn more calories throughout your day.

as hard as you can for 30 seconds, and you'll see what I mean!) But there's another surprising reason HIIT reshapes your belly.

The scientists who conducted the Australian study discovered that sprinting causes the body to release high levels of a group of hormones called *catecholamines,* which drive the release of abdominal and visceral fat. Senior study author Steve Boutcher said, "We don't know why, but moving limbs very fast generates high levels of catecholamine."[6]

This metabolic magic gives HIIT some serious belly-busting power. And because you get big results from a short exercise session, it's easy to work HIIT into even the busiest schedule.

The 10-Day Belly Slimdown HIIT Workout

To get you in the HIIT groove, I've asked fitness expert Natalie Jill to share ten simple but effective HIIT exercises you can do almost anywhere. In addition to being convenient, her workout is fast; the entire workout only takes 10 minutes!

To get started, simply perform the exercises below at a high intensity for 30 seconds with a 30-second rest in between each exercise. If you're new to HIIT or to exercising in general, start with five exercises and slowly work your way up to all ten.

According to Natalie, *intensity* and *progression* are the keys to your success, whether you work out for 5 minutes or 30 minutes—and whether you've never exercised in your life or you're a workout junkie. As you work out, keep these two tips in mind:

1. Perform each exercise at the highest intensity possible without compromising good form. When it comes to blasting belly fat, always keep your core engaged. Keep your ribs down, pull your ab muscles in, and squeeze your glutes.
2. Never stop challenging yourself. When you no longer break a sweat, take your workout to the next level. With HIIT, there are several ways to keep progressing:
   □ Repeat the circuit.

□ Increase your exercise time from 30 to 45 or 60 seconds.

□ Decrease your rest time from 30 to 20, 15, or 10 seconds.

High Knees

1. Stand up straight with your feet together.
2. Begin to jog in place, but raise your knees high toward your chest.
3. At the same time, pump your arms back and forth (in sync with your legs).

Plank Jacks

1. Start in a plank position with your arms fully extended. Keep your core engaged, and do not let your lower back sink down or arch at any time.
2. Jump your feet apart, back together, apart, and back together (similar to a jumping jack).

Jump Rope

Without actually using a jump rope, mimic jumping rope as fast as you can.

Knee to Elbow

1. Start in a plank position with your arms fully extended. Keep your core engaged, and do not let your lower back sink down or arch at any time.
2. Gently hop your right knee toward your right elbow.
3. Switch and gently hop your left knee toward your left elbow.
4. Keep alternating knees.

Shuffle Punch

1. Start in a standing position.
2. Shuffle your feet to the right three times, keeping your knees bent, and punch across your body in the direction you're traveling.

3. Shuffle back to the left three times and punch across your body in the direction you're traveling.
4. Keep alternating sides for 30 seconds.

Leapfrogs

1. Squat down into a frog position with your arms between your legs and your palms flat on the floor.
2. Jump your feet out behind you while keeping your core engaged. Then return to your starting position.
3. Your feet should come together when you jump out and then come back out to the sides of your arms when you jump in.

Butt Kicks

1. Start in a standing position with your feet together.
2. Bend your elbows and bring your arms into your chest at your sides for the entire exercise.
3. Kick your legs (one at a time) behind you and toward your butt, quickly alternating legs.

Jump Squats

1. Start in a standing position with your feet wider than shoulder width apart.
2. Squat down and press through the balls of your feet to jump up and out of your squat.

Soccer Toe Tap

1. Start in a standing position with your feet together.
2. Pretend there's a soccer ball in front of you. Tap your toe on the imaginary ball and continue alternating your feet and swinging your arms.

In and Outs

1. Start in plank position with your arms fully extended. Keep your core engaged, and do not let your lower back sink down at any time.
2. Jump both feet toward your chest, and then jump them back to the starting position.

Want a chance of pace? You can switch up the order of the exercises any time you want to keep things fresh.

Resistance Training

Resistance training, or strength training, means using weights—barbells, hand weights, or the weight of your own body—to create resistance that your muscles need to overcome. This is hard work, so you may want to postpone this type of exercise until you're done with your diet.

Resistance training is terrific for sculpting your core. (I call it "rearranging the furniture.") It helps you build lean muscle all over—

your butt, your thighs, your belly, the sides of your abdomen—and it pulls your gut up and in.

I know firsthand that resistance training will help you build a beautiful belly. That's because in my early twenties, I was into competitive body-building and even earned the title of Ms. St. Louis after winning one contest. (I was petite, but I was mighty!) My secret to looking amazing? Resistance training.

And don't worry—resistance training won't bulk you up. Instead, it will sculpt, strengthen, and tone your muscles. You won't get bulging muscles; you'll get sleek, sexy ones.

Resistance training has another big benefit, as well: It'll give you big results in a short time. Here's some of the research showing how fast it can work:

- Obese teens who did twelve weeks of strength training reduced their waist circumference and waist-to-hip ratio significantly.[8]

- In just six weeks, postmenopausal women reduced their fat mass, body mass index, percentage of body fat, and waist circumference through strength training.[9]

- In a study involving older men and women, twelve weeks of resistance training led to decreases in waist circumference, visceral fat thickness, and thigh fat thickness.[10]

One of the biggest keys to resistance training is to keep challenging your muscles. To do this, start with the heaviest weights you can lift *safely with good form*. Over time, increase the amount of weight you use, and shorten the time between your repetitions.

Now, it may surprise you, but I want you to do resistance training only *every other day*. The reason for this is that your muscles need a full day to rest, restore, and rebuild themselves.

When you do a resistance workout, you actually create microscopic tears in your muscles. I know this sounds bad, but it's actually a very good thing. Your body reacts to the damage by rebuilding your muscles, making them stronger in the process. This remodeling job is every bit as important as the exercise itself, so you need those days off.

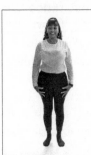
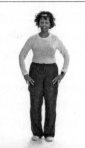

BEFORE   AFTER

CLARE VALDRAY

WEIGHT LOST: 8.4 POUNDS | HIP INCHES LOST: 2.5 | THIGH INCHES LOST: .75

Clare is one of our most successful losers, despite the fact that she's over sixty. (She doesn't look it, does she?) Clare actually lost the most weight on her hips, thighs, and bust, which is where she needed to lose it.

After she finished her diet, Clare told me, "I was amazed at the fact that I had no appetite whatsoever . . . no cravings, nothing. Usually after I work a full day, I'm ready to eat a meal. But I went ten hours and got home and did a shake, and I noticed, 'I'm not hungry.' After the shake, I knew I had to wait again, and I still wasn't hungry."

She added, "I felt like I had more energy . . . and I just kept saying, 'I don't have an appetite.' I could go past restaurants and not feel like I had to turn in to the restaurant. I [usually] have a chocolate craving, and I didn't crave chocolate."

When I asked Clare if she'd recommend the 10-Day Belly Slimdown to other people, she laughed and said, "I already have. I have three people on board already." As for Clare, now that she's kick-started her weight loss, she's planning to take off still more pounds by transitioning to my 21-Day Bone Broth Diet.

The 10-Day Belly Slimdown Resistance Workout

Here's a quick, easy, core-shaping workout—also designed by my buddy Natalie Jill—that you can do at home using just your body weight.

Simply perform the exercises as described with a 30-second rest in between each. And don't forget about intensity and progression! Keep your core engaged, and give each exercise your all. Once the workout gets easier, progress: Perform the exercises longer, rest for less time, or repeat the circuit.

Bridge Ladder

1. Start by lying on your back, knees bent, feet flat on the floor, and your arms by your sides.
2. Lift your hips into a bridge position and hold for 1–2 seconds.
3. Bring your hips back down to starting position.
4. Repeat for 30 seconds.

Wall Sits

1. Press your back against a wall and carefully lower yourself to nearly a "sitting" position, with your feet out in front of you and your knees at a 90-degree angle.
2. Reach your arms straight ahead of you for balance.
3. Hold this position for 30 to 60 seconds.

Lean-Backs

1. Start on your knees with your arms clasped in front of you.
2. Engage your core and glute muscles to make sure you do not strain your back.
3. Lean back and hold this position for 30 seconds.

Frog Touch Down to Stand Up

1. Start standing up straight.
2. Drop down into a frog position with your knees out wide and your arms between your legs.

3. Stand back up, engaging your glutes and triceps.
4. Repeat for 30 seconds.

Tabletop

1. Sit on your bottom with your knees bent and feet together. Place your hands about a foot behind your bottom, with your palms flat on the floor and your fingers pointing toward your toes.
2. Lift your hips to make a flat "table" with your torso.
3. Hold this position for 30 seconds.

Donkey Kicks

1. On your forearms and knees, lift your right leg behind you at a 90-degree angle. Keep your foot flat and flexed and push it toward the ceiling. Engage your core and squeeze your hamstrings and glutes.
2. Do as many lifts as you can in 30 seconds.
3. Switch sides and repeat for 30 seconds.

Explosive Wall Push-Ups

1. Stand 10 to 12 inches more than arm's length away from a wall. With your arms straight, lean toward the wall, keeping your body straight, and place your palms flat on the wall.
2. Bend your elbows to move your upper body toward the wall as if you were doing a push-up. Your elbows should be pointing down and not out to the side.
3. Push off the wall with full force, then return to the starting position.
4. Repeat for 30 seconds.

Chair (or Sofa) Sit

1. Start out in a standing position about a foot in front of a very stable chair or sofa, facing out. Lift your arms straight out in front of you. Engage your core. Keep your shoulders back and your chin and chest up to help with balance.
2. Drop down into a sitting position with your knees at a 90-degree angle.

3. As you stand back up, push through your heels, engaging your glutes.
4. Repeat for 30 seconds.

Sumo Squat

1. Start with your feet slightly wider than shoulder width apart. Engage your core.
2. Squat low to engage your glutes and legs.
3. Push through your heels on your way up.
4. Repeat for 30 seconds.

Walk-Outs to a Push-Up

1. In a standing position, reach your palms down to the floor and "walk" your hands out until you're in a push-up position.
2. Do a push-up and "walk" your hands back to the starting position while engaging your core.
3. Repeat for 30 seconds.

Bonus Workouts

I asked Natalie (who has killer abs, by the way) to share her absolute favorite core workouts. Start with the basic workout, and add the "Advanced Sexy Core Plank Challenge" as you get stronger.

The 10-Day Belly Slimdown Bonus Core Workout

Perform the exercises with intensity as described below with 30 seconds of rest between each. Keep challenging yourself to achieve the best results.

For the plank exercises, intensity is all about form. Holding a plank for 60 seconds isn't effective unless your abs are pulled in, your back is flat, and your glutes are squeezed.

Plank

1. Start out in a standard plank position on your forearms and toes (with your hands clasped together).
2. Keep your hips lifted and core engaged to prevent your lower back from sinking down or arching up.
3. Hold this position for 30 to 60 seconds.

Side Plank

1. Start by lying on your right side on the floor.
2. Resting on your right forearm with your legs outstretched, lift your hips to create a straight line from your head to your toes.
3. Keep your core engaged, not letting your hips drop.
4. Hold this position for 30 to 60 seconds.
5. Switch sides and hold for 30 to 60 seconds.

Pike Walkouts

1. Start in a push-up position. Engage your core.
2. Walk your feet toward your hands, remembering to contract your ab muscles.
3. Walk your feet back out.
4. Repeat for 60 seconds.

V Holds

1. Start out lying on your back and stretch your arms out over your head and parallel to the floor with your fingertips pointing toward the wall behind you.
2. Lift your legs and bring your arms and legs toward each other to create a V position with your body.
3. Contract your abdominal muscles and hold for 15 to 30 seconds.

Shimmies—Flat Back, Shimmy Side to Side

1. Lie flat on your back with your knees bent and feet flat on the floor. Slightly lift your shoulders with your chin tucked in. Keep

the rest of your back flat on the floor, with your arms by your sides and your palms facing down.

2. "Shimmy" your right fingertips to touch your right heel and back, then shimmy your left fingertips to touch your left heel, keeping your motion continuous.

3. Continue alternating sides for 60 seconds.

Flutter Kicks

1. Lie on your back with your legs outstretched, raise your upper back, and rest on your forearms/elbows. Engage your core.

2. Elevate your feet, engage your core, and crisscross or "flutter kick" your feet back and forth over each other.

3. Continue flutter kicking for 30 seconds.

Flat Back Hand to Foot

1. Lying on your back with your legs and arms outstretched, simultaneously raise your right hand and your left foot to touch straight above you, slightly lifting your head.

2. Switch sides to raise your left hand and your right foot to touch.

3. Continue alternating sides for 60 seconds.

Slow Bicycles

1. Lie on your back with your legs outstretched, raise your upper back, and rest on your forearms/elbows.

2. Pull your legs one at a time toward your chest in a bicycle pedaling motion for 60 seconds.

V Ups and Downs

This is similar to the V Hold. In the V Hold, you hold the position. In V Ups and Downs, you form the V, return to your starting position, and then form the V again.

1. Lie on your back with your arms extended above your head and your legs lifted at a 45-degree angle. Engage your core.

2. Bring your arms and legs toward each other into a V position while contracting your abs.

3. Return to the starting position and repeat for 60 seconds.

Up and Down Scissor Kicks

1. Lie on your back with your legs outstretched.
2. Elevate your feet, pressing your lower back into the floor.
3. Move your straight legs up and down in a "scissors" motion.
4. Continue alternating legs for 30 seconds.

Advanced Sexy-Core Plank Challenge

For this advanced plank challenge, perform each exercise as described, resting for 30 seconds in between each one.

Side Plank Walks

1. Start in a side plank position, with your weight on your right hand.
2. Walk your feet forward and back for 30 seconds.
3. Switch sides, with your left hand on the floor, and walk your feet forward and back for 30 seconds.

High Plank, Knee to Opposite Twist

1. Start in a push-up/plank position with your arms fully extended.
2. Bring your right knee in toward your opposite wrist. Hold for a second.
3. Repeat for 30 seconds and then switch sides.

Side Plank Hold with Leg Up

1. Start in a side plank position on your forearm.
2. Lift your top leg and hold this position for 30 seconds. If you can, also extend your arm upward toward the ceiling to increase the difficulty.
3. Repeat on the other side for 30 seconds.

Up Up Down Down

1. Start in a standard plank position on your forearms.
2. Lift your right forearm off the floor, and then place your right hand where your forearm was.
3. Repeat with your left arm, so you're now in a plank/push-up position on your hands rather than your forearms.

4. Lower your body weight back onto your forearms, starting with your right side first and following with your left side.
5. Repeat for 30 seconds.
6. Perform a second cycle for 30 seconds, starting with the opposite side.

Side Plank with Hip Dips

1. Start in a side plank on your right forearm.
2. Lift your hips up and drop them down toward the floor, engaging your core the entire time.
3. Repeat for 30 seconds.
4. Switch sides and repeat for 30 seconds.

Bird Dogs from Hands and Feet

1. Start in a plank/push-up position with your arms fully extended.
2. Reach your right arm out while lifting your left leg off the ground at the same time. Hold for 2 seconds.
3. Repeat, starting on the other side, reaching your left arm out and right leg off the ground.
4. Continue alternating arms and legs for 30 seconds.

Side Plank Knee to Elbow

1. Start in a side plank position on your right forearm with your left arm over your head.
2. Bring your elbow and your left knee together while engaging your core.
3. Return to the starting position and repeat for 30 seconds.
4. Switch sides and repeat for 30 seconds.

Plank—Side-to-Side Toe Tap

1. Start in a standard plank position on your forearms.
2. Tap your left toe out to the side at about a 45-degree angle and return to the starting position.
3. Tap your right toe out to the side and return to the starting position.
4. Continue alternating sides for 30 seconds.

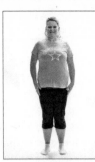
BEFORE

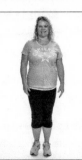
AFTER

MARY DORR

WEIGHT LOST: 4.6 POUNDS | BELLY INCHES LOST: 1.5

Even though she confesses to cheating, Mary lost nearly five pounds on the 10-Day Belly Slimdown. "I haven't been under two hundred pounds in more than twenty-five years," she says. "It renews your motivation and your commitment."

If you give in to temptation and have a cheat or two, don't sweat it. Like Mary, you'll still lose weight. And if you want to lose the maximum amount of belly fat, you can simply take a break for a day or two and then start your ten-day program over again.

Hand Plank Reaches

1. Start in a plank/push-up position with your arms fully extended.
2. Reach your left hand out as far ahead of you as you can; then bring it back to starting position.
3. Do the same with your right hand.
4. Continue alternating sides for 30 seconds.

Plank Knee to Same Side Elbow

1. Start in a standard plank position on your forearms.
2. Bring your right knee out to the side to meet your right elbow and return to the starting position.

3. Bring your left knee out to the side to meet your left elbow and return to the starting position.

4. Continue alternating sides for 30 seconds.

EASY HACKS FOR "REARRANGING THE FURNITURE"

In addition to diet and exercise, here are five magic tricks that can make your belly look smaller (or, in the case of the fifth one, even make it smaller for real):

- Get rid of "purse pooch." According to cosmetic surgeon Michael Prager, women pack extra fat onto their bodies when they carry oversize, overstuffed handbags. Posture expert Ivana Daniell says that's because a postural imbalance affects how you distribute fat.[11] The solution? Pack less stuff in your bag, switch it frequently from one side to the other, or switch out a big handbag for something smaller.

- Stand up straight. If you spend your days slouched in front of a computer or hunched over your phone, you're wrecking your posture—and bad posture makes your belly look fatter. Get in the habit of standing tall, on the other hand, and you'll look slimmer—plus, you'll make your neck, shoulders, and knees happier and allow your lungs to take in more oxygen.

- To improve your posture, try the "string" trick: When you're standing or walking, imagine that there's a string fastened to the top of your head, pulling you gently upward. (Practice this standing sideways in front of a mirror, and you'll be amazed at the difference it makes.)

- Buy a better bra. Most women aren't wearing a bra that fits well. A good bra lifts your bust, making you look slimmer because there's more distance between your hips and your chest.

- Try an infrared sauna. Research, though preliminary, suggests that using an infrared sauna can reduce your waist circumference.[12] See if your local gym has one—and if so, give it a try.

Keep Slimming Your Belly on Your "Off" Days

Earlier, I said that you don't need to exercise on your diet days. However, this doesn't mean that you should just sit on your butt on those days. Even if you're battling the "carb flu" (see page 71), I want you to get off that couch and move!

By now, you've probably heard that "sitting is the new smoking," and it's true. Sitting for hours is incredibly bad for your body. It lowers your metabolism, puts belly fat on you, increases your risk of metabolic syndrome, and even ups your risk for cancer.

So don't spend your diet days parked on your behind. At work, get up every 15 minutes and do some stretches or take a walk around the office. At home, weed the garden, toss a ball for the dog, or take a walk or an easy bike ride. All these activities will boost your metabolism, melting off more fat.

One of my rules for a healthy life is that you need to move for at least one hour every day. You don't need to knock yourself out—any kind of activity you enjoy is fine. The important thing is to just *get up and get going* every chance you get. The more you move your body, the leaner, shapelier, and healthier your belly will be . . . it truly is that simple!

SHRINK YOUR WAIST BY BUSTING YOUR STRESS

know you're focused on a short-term goal right now: getting a gorgeous, sexy belly *fast*. And that's what the next ten days are all about. Together, we're going to slash your belly fat.

But let me tell you the same thing I tell my clients:

I can take that bulge off your belly right now—but the only way you'll keep it off is if you get control over your stress. If you don't do this, I can guarantee that your flat belly will turn back into flab.

Why do I say this? Because if chronic stress takes control of your life, it will take control of your belly, too. Here's what that stress does to you:

- It causes you to urgently crave sugar and fat. (That's because your stress hormones are *made* of sugar and fat.) So you're going reach for the foods that put that fat on you in the first place.

- It raises your cortisol levels, and cortisol packs on fat around your waist. As a result, you'll wind up with a "cortisol tire"—that belly roll you see even on many skinny people.

There's no way I'm going to let this happen on my watch. I don't want you to take that fat off only to put it right back on! So right now, we need to talk about the next step in the 10-Day Belly Slimdown: *getting that stress under control.*

Yes—You Can!

I know you may be thinking, "Get real, Dr. Kellyann." If you spend every day running like your hair's on fire—juggling a job, a home, volunteer work, maybe even kids—you may think I'm nuts to even *suggest* that you can take charge of your stress.

But you know what? The celebrities I work with have crazy lives, too. They're on stages or movie sets for hours at a time. They're memorizing lines, recording songs, promoting albums, and somehow squeezing in a personal life—all while trying to keep the paparazzi at bay. Even with an entourage of people to help them out, they're always on the run. Still, my techniques empower them to cut their stress down to size.

So hear me out. No matter how crazy your life is, you can do this. What's more, you *need* to do it. It's not optional . . . it's *necessary.*

And I'm not simply saying that as a professional. You see, I learned this the hard way myself.

How Stress Brought Me Down . . . and How I Fought Back

I'm a weight-loss and anti-aging expert, and I know my stuff. But a decade ago, I hit a low point. I'd helped thousands of people get fit and younger looking, but for once, I didn't know how to help myself.

I was just entering my forties—that time when so many of us, especially women, "hit the wall" between young and old.

And that's exactly what I did. I hit that wall *hard*—like a semi-truck going ninety miles an hour.

I was burned out, gaining weight, and getting a "cortisol tire." My hair started thinning. I was moody all the time. I call it my "fat, bitchy, and bald" period.

I remember seeing my reflection in the door of a freezer case at the store and not even recognizing myself because I looked so *old*. I thought, "OMG. *This cannot be happening.*"

My health and my looks depended on my getting my groove back. And so did my career—because nothing says *failure* like a weight-loss and anti-aging expert who's starting to look like a wrinkled Teletubby.

So I took stock. What was I doing wrong? I took a long, hard look at my lifestyle. And pretty quickly, I identified the problem.

At the time, I was raising two young boys while writing five books and working full-time at my clinic. I was spending all my remaining hours doing volunteer work, sharing my message on TV and radio, ferrying my kids to baseball games, and trying to keep up with the laundry.

It was too much. And I was paying the price.

While I was spending my days telling people how to get slim and fit, I was spending my evenings eating starchy comfort foods. While I was telling people to value themselves, I was neglecting my own needs.

My life was spiraling out of control, and I knew that I needed a drastic change. So I took control—first, by reducing my stress and then by learning how to cope with it. And in just a minute, I'm going to tell you how to do the same thing.

First, however, I want you to take a closer look at the toll that stress is taking on you—not just in terms of your weight, but in terms of your life. Here's a quiz that can help you see how much stress is impacting your life.

Do you feel, every day or almost every day, as if you have to keep running at top speed to get everything done?

Do you frequently wake up in the middle of the night stressing over work issues, family issues, or other problems?

Do you frequently find yourself reaching for such foods as ice cream, pizza, potato chips, or macaroni and cheese when you're stressed?

Do you often have trouble concentrating because you feel stressed?

Do you often experience headaches, backaches, or digestive upsets?

Do you have a hard time enjoying leisure activities because you're constantly thinking about things you need to be doing?

Do you often snap at your family members because you feel overwhelmed?

Do you drink more alcohol than you should?

Do you feel older than you are?

Are you both wired and tired all the time?

If you said yes to many or most of these questions, then chronic stress has you firmly in its clutches—and *it's time to fight back*. Here's how to do it.

Step 1: Strategize Your Yesses

If you're a good person at heart, I'm betting that you have a very hard time saying no when someone asks you to take on an obligation. And you know what I have to say about that?

Get over it.

This was the biggest secret I had to learn when I hit the wall. When I took a step back and looked at my life, I realized that I was exhausting myself doing things for other people and spending zero time doing things for myself.

That's when I realized that I needed to start being *strategic* about my time. So I began asking myself these questions every time someone asked me to take on a new responsibility:

- If I say yes, what am I really agreeing to? How much work will it involve? Is it worth that much work?

- If I say yes, what effect will my decision have on my family, my own life, and my work?

- If I say yes, will I be violating any of my core values—for instance, my belief that I need to follow a healthy lifestyle?

I'm not exaggerating when I say that this strategy didn't just take years off my face and pounds off my belly; it changed my life. It gave me time for the things I love, from doing ballet to puttering in the kitchen to hanging out with my sons. For the first time in ages, I could stop running and just *be*.

And it's not just me who's benefited. People who've read *Dr. Kellyann's Bone Broth Diet*—where I first talked about strategizing your yesses—tell me over and over again that doing this has changed their lives, too. I firmly believe that it will do the same thing for you.

And by the way, while you're strategizing your yesses when it comes to obligations, start doing the same thing when it comes to relationships. I call this "having an inner doorman." It's great to be *friendly* with everyone, but be *friends* only with a small inner circle of people who bring positive energy into your life. These are the people who will reduce your stress, rather than increasing it.

Step 2: Become Stress-Resilient

You can minimize the stress in your life by strategizing your yesses, but you'll never get *rid* of that stress entirely. There's always some-

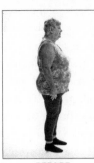

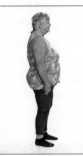

BEFORE   AFTER

SANDY CARPENTER

WEIGHT LOST: 10 POUNDS | BELLY INCHES LOST: 2.75

Sandy, a sugar freak, wasn't at all sure she could go for ten days without a candy fix. She told her neighbor Mary, who did the diet with her (see Mary's success story on page 187), "In about five days, you'd better come check on me and make sure I'm not in a coma from not having sugar."

To her happy surprise, Sandy was able to do the whole ten days without a single cheat—and with almost no cravings! And she's ecstatic about her ten-pound weight loss, which equates to a pound per day. Awesome—especially for someone at the age of sixty-three.

---

thing to worry about—your job, your family, your health, your never-ending bills.

Also, life loves to hit you with sucker punches. One day, it's a flat tire on the freeway. The next day, it's a rumor about layoffs, or the discovery that your daughter's dating a punk rocker with purple hair and a Satan tattoo.

Unfortunately, you can't simply say, "No thanks, life. I'm returning this day to you—please send me a better one." However, you *can* take steps to stress-proof yourself when life is crazy. Here are some of the most powerful ways to stay strong, centered, and calm when everything's going to hell in a handbasket.

Do mindful meditation. I know lots of people think that meditation is just a "Hollywood thing" or something that aging hippies do. But in reality, people have used meditation for centuries—and now science is revealing just how effective it is at relieving stress.

For instance, research shows that a simple, eight-week meditation program can actually *change the structure of your brain* in ways that foster emotional control.[1] In addition, the deep breathing you do while meditating triggers that powerful "relaxation response" I talked about in the previous chapter.

And meditation isn't just effective—it's also simple, although it takes practice to do it easily. Here are the steps.

- Find a quiet place where no one will interrupt you. (If all else fails, lock yourself in the bathroom.)

- Get into a comfortable position in a chair or on the floor. Rest your hands lightly on your thighs. Close your eyes if you'd like.

- Notice how you feel. Are you tired? Cool? Warm? Are you experiencing any tension or pain in any part of your body? How does your clothing feel against your skin?

- Notice your surroundings. What do you hear or smell?

- Let your mind wander where it will. At first, it will probably be swirling with thoughts about work, money, or family issues. That's okay. Simply examine each thought without judging it, and then gently let it go.

- Focus on your breathing. Take deep breaths in, as if you're filling your abdomen with air. Then slowly let each breath out. Focusing on your breathing helps you stay anchored as you meditate. When your mind wanders, let it—and then return your attention to your breathing.

- If it helps to relax you further, say a soothing word or sound as you breathe out.

If you're new to meditation, be patient, because it takes a while to get the hang of it. The more you practice, the easier it'll become.

HAPPINESS AND BELLY FAT

ELIZABETH LOMBARDO, PHD

Clinical psychologist, speaker, and coach

Bestselling author of *A Happy You: Your Ultimate Prescription for Happiness* and *Better than Perfect: 7 Strategies to Crush Your Inner Critic and Create a Life You Love*

Facebook @Dr.Elizabeth.Lombardo

ElizabethLombardo.com

People often think, "I'll be happier *when . . .*" as in, "I'll be happier *when* I lose my belly fat." But did you know that the opposite is actually true? No, I don't mean you will be sadder when you lose the weight. I mean that being happier *now* can actually help you lose the belly fat.

When you are feeling happy, you experience less stress. In fact, research shows that when people experience gratitude (a key component of happiness), the stress centers in their brain reduce their activity, so they feel less stressed. And stress can prevent you from losing belly fat.

How? A few ways, really. First, biologically, stress adversely impacts your body. From interfering with your digestive system to causing fat to be laid down in the abdomen, stress works against all the hard work you are doing applying Dr. Kellyann's wisdom.

Second, stress can impact our actions. Think of stress as being on a continuum from 0 (no stress at all) to 10 (the most stressed you've ever been). When we get to higher levels of stress, 7–10 or more, we tend to think in more negative ways and act in less healthy ways. I call it the Red Zone when you are at a 7–10 on the stress scale. And I coach my clients, "Don't let anything out of your mouth (say something you may later regret) or put anything into your mouth (eat what you may later regret) when you are in the Red Zone."

Third, stress interferes with sleep. Maybe you can relate. Despite how exhausted you might be, when your head hits the pillow, your mind starts racing and keeping you up. Or maybe you can fall asleep, but in the middle of the night that stressed mind starts chatting up a storm, and you can't turn it off. Well, not getting the sleep you need is associated with gaining more weight. So your fatigue may be contributing to your belly fat.

Luckily, you do not have to be a victim of your stress. You can control your stress and be happy right now. Here are some of the strategies you can try today:

1. **Write a thank-you note.** Gratitude is a great way to reduce stress and feel happier. You can do this by focusing on what and whom you appreciate, even keeping this list in a gratitude journal. Another way to feel more gratitude is by writing a thank-you note. This note is not in reaction to a birthday gift you may have received, but rather to someone in your past who gave you an intangible gift. Perhaps it was a teacher who gave you a boost of confidence that you continue to carry around or an old friend who was there for you when you really needed him or her. Just grab a pen and paper and start sharing what you appreciate about that person, what they taught you, how grateful you are for what they did. It doesn't have to be perfect (see #3), just heartfelt and sincere. Should you send it? That is up to you. You will feel happier just writing it. And imagine the joy you could bring to that person if they actually heard this gratitude from you. (Bonus: Acts of kindness also boost the happiness of the person doing those acts, so this could be a double happiness booster.)

2. **Give yourself a time-out (*before* you need it).** The antidote for selfishness is not selflessness. You are not a better person if you only focus on the needs of others. You *are* stressed out, though. Taking time for yourself is not being self-centered; it is being smart. Take time for yourself each day to do something that brings *you* positive energy. Maybe it is a 10-minute walk in nature, 5 minutes of meditation, or even a few extra minutes in a warm shower. Or it could be something bigger, like splurging on a massage or going to see a funny movie. Taking time for yourself will not only help you be happier, but will also help you be a better you (parent, partner, caregiver, worker, etc.).

3. **Drop the perfectionism.** Perfectionism is way more than just liking the junk drawer to be neat. It is an all-or-nothing mentality: Something is either perfect or it's a failure. Perfectionism can interfere with your happiness ("I made a mistake; I am such a failure"), your health ("I had one cookie and messed up my diet, might as well eat the rest of the plate"), your relationships ("He didn't ask me how my day was; he doesn't care about me"), and your work ("I am afraid I won't get the promotion, so I am not going to even try"). Do you see the all-or-nothing, perfect-or-failure, perfect-or-forget-it mind-set here? The goal is to drop the stressful parts of perfectionism and be "Better Than Perfect."

When you are a happier you, your belly will be happier, too, and it will drop some of its fat. Give these strategies a try today.

Try yoga or Tai Chi. I'm betting that you're already familiar with yoga, which involves breathing control and physical poses designed to increase flexibility, reduce tension, and improve strength and balance. Tai Chi, an ancient form of exercise involving slow, ballet-like movements, has similar benefits.

Both yoga and Tai Chi are forms of "moving meditation," and science shows that they're powerful stress-busters. For instance:

- One study followed emotionally distressed women, half of whom were asked to participate in twice-weekly yoga sessions. At the end of three months, depression scores improved by 50%, anxiety scores by 30%, and overall well-being scores by 65% in the yoga group.[2]

- A meta-analysis studying the effects of Tai Chi reviewed data from 40 studies and concluded, "Tai Chi appears to be associated with improvements in psychological well-being including reduced stress, anxiety, depression and mood disturbance, and increased self-esteem."[3]

THE CONFIDENCE-BELLY FAT CONNECTION

SHARON MELNICK, PHD

Bestselling author of *Success Under Stress: Powerful Tools for Staying Calm, Confident, and Productive When the Pressure's On* and *Confidence When It Counts: Rise Above Self-Criticism and Bias to Make Your Mark*

SharonMelnick.com

What does confidence have to do with belly fat? Low self-confidence causes stress, stress raises cortisol, and cortisol sets up cravings that can accumulate belly fat.

When you lack confidence, your brain will always make you do something to deal with that issue before it will let you take action on your longer-term health goals. People who successfully lose and keep weight off have been shown to have a "meditative element" in their lives. They are intentional—able to confidently act in the service of what they want.

Here are five ways your confidence affects your belly fat, along with tips to show up for life confidently:

1. CONFIDENCE HELPS YOU BE IN YOUR POWER—NOT REACT.

In response to a difficult person, do you get hijacked by a wave of negative emotion? Do you either feel angry and disrespected ("He's a jerk!") or take the provocation personally ("I'm not good enough")? If so, you may be tempted to satisfy these emotional states through food (e.g., crunch on chips to relieve anger, soothe yourself with ice cream).

Tip: Source your confidence from within, so you can care about other people but not so much about what you think their actions are saying about you. Be impeccable with your 50%—what you bring—in any interaction. Recognize that the other person likely is being difficult because he or she is limited. Stop giving away your power. Accept the other person's level of evolution, and work on your own!

2. CONFIDENCE CREATES ENERGY STATES IN YOUR BODY.

Scientists guesstimate that human beings have about 60,000 thoughts a day. Every thought has an energetic consequence—it either lights you up and brings joy or drags you down and creates stress. It doesn't take days or weeks to feel great in your body; you have 60,000 opportunities a day to build the energy state you want.

Tip: Ask yourself, "Who do I need to be in order to create the results I want? What are the qualities and attributes of the person I need to show up as?" Come up with a phrase that describes that "horizon point" (e.g., *Confident Leader*, *Calm Appreciator*). You may not be able to instantly create all the change and success you want, but you *can* instantly become the person you need to be to create them.

3. CONFIDENCE DETERMINES YOUR FOCUS.

Doubt and judgment focus on your momentary concerns: "How can I fade into the curtains in this situation?" or "I'm not good enough" or "How can I get this person to treat me better?" These concerns are your "small game." Instead, play your "big game"!

Tip: Your small game consists of the ways in which you try to control others to get love. Instead, *be* love! What's the contribution you want to make while you are in this life? Whom do you want to help, and what is the legacy you want to leave? Instead of hiding, go to the party! Talk about things you are passionate about, and bring a big smile that lights up the room. It's the fastest way to be beautiful, and you will magnetize people around you.

4. CONFIDENCE MAKES YOU CONSTRUCTIVE AND COMPASSIONATE.

Confidence is about the way you make a relationship with yourself. Low self-confidence makes you lose touch with yourself: You either beat yourself up with regret about the past or live in fear of what will happen. Self-compassion brings you back to the present moment.

Tip: If you do something that you didn't want to do, be a detective. Use self-compassion as a bridge from the negativity rabbit hole to seeing what happened as something you can understand and, thus, do differently next time. "What was going on that led me to do that? How can I see this as only one moment of my whole life of goodness?"

5. KNOW YOUR CONFIDENCE TYPE.

Confidence is not "one size fits all." Find out your type, and source your confidence in a way that's right for your type.

If you seek approval, find an activity that will help you feel filled up from within (for instance, meditation, gardening, or reading) instead of relying on the validation of others.

If you hold back, shift your question from "Who am I to speak up or go for a bigger life?" to "What value can I bring to others?"

If you are a perfectionist, work hard, but practice 5 minutes of deep breathing each day. It will calm your brain enough that you can gain perspective on the reality of how good you really are, what you *really want* (as opposed to what you feel obliged to do), and what's most important to you (such as making space to be present with the people you really love).

As a plus, yoga and Tai Chi won't just de-stress you. In addition, either one will also give you a good exercise workout that will count toward that hour of movement I want you to work in every day. It's another of those "two-fers" that I love!

If you're new to yoga, I recommend starting with hatha yoga or a similar gentle version. (Challenging forms, such as Bikram or Ashtanga yoga, may stress you out rather than relaxing you.) Also, experiment with different classes and different teachers, and see which is the best match for you.

If you have back problems or other health conditions that could make any form of yoga difficult, Tai Chi is a great alternative. It requires less strength and balance, and it's easier on your joints and muscles.

Evaluate your stressors. If your stress is maxing out the meter, have a heart-to-heart discussion with yourself about what's causing it, what you can do about it, and what you *want* to do about it. Make a list of your stressors, and make a decision to accept the things you can't change, and avoid, eliminate, or alleviate the others. For instance, if you have a family member you find stressful to be around, consider seeing that person less frequently.

Get a massage, treat yourself to "float therapy," or take an Epsom salt bath. There's nothing like a massage to blitz stress and leave you feeling all warm and fuzzy—unless it's flotation therapy, which is also hugely popular these days. In float therapy, you lie in a light- and soundproof cocoon filled with water so loaded with Epsom salts that you actually float. The sensory deprivation, the magnesium you absorb, and the relaxation of floating (which eases aches and pains) can leave you feeling mellow for hours or even days afterward.

Of course, massages and float therapy might not fit into your budget right now. If not, you can get the same relaxing benefits by taking an Epsom salt bath in the evening. Simply add 2 cups of Epsom salt to your bathwater (along with some essential oils, if you have them). Spend at least half an hour in the tub, so the magnesium in the Epsom salt can soothe and relax you. You'll dial that stress way down, and you'll sleep like a baby.

Consider acupuncture. Acupuncture isn't just helpful for pain; it can also reduce stress. Acupuncture can cause your body temperature to go down; your organ systems, heartbeat, and respiration to slow down; and your muscle tension to dissipate. All of this can ease you into a very relaxed state.

Journal. Are you a nighttime worrier? Do you have trouble falling asleep or wake up at 2:00 a.m. and start fretting over your problems?

If so, take 5 or 10 minutes *before* bedtime each night to write about the things that are troubling you. In addition, take time to write about the good things in your life. This will help you put things in perspective—and often, it'll help you think of solutions to your problems. As a result, you'll doze off more quickly and spend less time tossing and turning.

Also, consider making a to-do list before bedtime. This will help keep your mind uncluttered after you turn in for the night.

Get more sleep. I know it's tempting to skimp on ZZZZ's in order to cross a few more stressful chores off your list. But when you deprive yourself of sleep, you're going to feel even *more* stressed out the next day. That's because a sleep deficit leads to "brain fog," making that to-do list an even bigger mountain to climb.

What's more, you'll be doing your belly a big favor if you get to

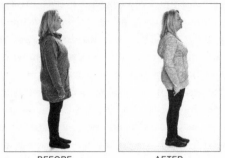

BEFORE   AFTER

LINDA RAFFERTY

WEIGHT LOST: 6.4 POUNDS | BELLY INCHES LOST: 4

One of the biggest surprises for Linda on the diet was that her chronic back and ankle pain disappeared. In addition to loving her slimmer waist, she's enjoying what she calls a "generalized great feeling"!

bed on time. That's because sleep can make you slimmer by cutting your food cravings down to size.

In one intriguing study,[4] researchers asked volunteers to participate in two experiments. In the first, the participants spent eight and a half hours in bed each night for four days. In the second, they spent only four and a half hours in bed each night for four days. Participants ate identical meals on both occasions.

The researchers measured participants' levels of a chemical signal called 2-AG, which enhances the pleasure of eating. They predicted that sleep deprivation would activate 2-AG, making people hungrier—and it turned out they were right.

When participants slept longer, their 2-AG levels stayed low in the morning, peaked after lunch, and dropped as the day went on. But when the participants slept less, their 2-AG levels rose to levels 33% higher than normal, peaking at 2:00 p.m. and staying high until about 9:00 p.m.

The sleep-deprived participants reported being hungrier around the time their 2-AG levels peaked. In addition, they craved high-calorie snacks, even after a big meal.

In short, cheating yourself on sleep can cost you dearly the next day—not just by stressing you out, but also by messing with your hunger signals and making you crazy for the foods that go straight to your belly.

Want still another reason to get more sleep? In separate research, scientists found that people who suffer from sleep deprivation (less than six hours of sleep per night) are nearly five times more likely to progress from normal blood sugar levels to impaired fasting glucose, compared to people who sleep for six to eight hours per night.[5] So getting good sleep won't just make you slimmer; it'll also reduce your risk for diabetes.

Clearly, if you want to banish that belly fat for good, it's a smart idea to stop burning the candle at both ends. I know this isn't easy, but here are some tricks that can help you succeed:

- Set a bedtime for yourself, and stick to it as closely as you can. Regular bedtimes aren't just for the kiddos—they're crucial for grown-ups, too!

- Turn off your phone and other devices, and tell your friends not to call you within half an hour of your bedtime. The blue light projected by your devices messes with your levels of melatonin (a hormone that helps control your sleep-wake cycles), making it harder for you to doze off and stay asleep. And here's still another reason to put that phone down: Research shows that evening exposure to the blue light from devices makes you hungry and promotes insulin resistance—so it's directly contributing to your belly fat![6]

- If you just can't tear yourself away from your devices after dark, look into purchasing some blue light–blocking glasses. They're fairly inexpensive, and they can help you sleep after a night of texting or surfing.

- Create a bedtime ritual. Taking a bath, dimming the lights, playing the same soft music each night, and even rubbing a touch of lavender onto your bed's headboard can trigger your brain to be ready for sleep. A little yoga, meditation, or stretching can relax you, as well. However, don't do strenuous exercise within three hours of bedtime; it will raise your body temperature and cause you to be more alert, making it hard to doze off.

- Keep your room dark and the temperature cool—between 60 and 66 degrees.

- Invest in quality bedding, and replace pillows yearly and your mattress every seven years.

- Consider creating a "time-free" zone in your bedroom. If you need an alarm clock, place it out of sight.

- Limit how much you eat and drink before bedtime. If you want a drink, chose water or herbal tea rather than coffee or alcohol.

As a general rule, aim for at least seven hours of sleep per night. That will help you awaken rested and refreshed each day—and as the research shows, it may also take inches off your waistline.

So if it's late at night, and you're reading this book, do yourself a favor . . . put it down right now, and *go to bed!*

P.S. One of the best biomarkers of adequate sleep is the a.m. cortisol test. Cortisol is the "get up and go" hormone. It should be nice and high when you wake up and gently go down as the day progresses. If your a.m. cortisol test is low, it can indicate a major sleep disturbance such as obstructive sleep apnea. You can get your a.m. cortisol as well as other hormones tested at YourLabWork.com/Dr-Kellyann.

Have a giggle. It's not just a cliché; laughter really *is* good medicine. It stimulates your heart and lungs, causes your body to release happy-making endorphins, and relaxes your muscles. So when you're stressed, take a 10-minute time-out to listen to a comedy skit, read a funny book, or call a friend who makes you laugh.

Make a "gratitude" list. It's easy to lose sight of the good things in your life when you're battling rush-hour traffic, worrying about money, or calling the plumber after your toddler flushed his sis-

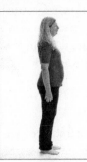
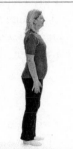

BEFORE   AFTER

FRAN TATARELLI

WEIGHT LOST: 7 POUNDS (AFTER LOSING 40+ POUNDS ON THE ORIGINAL BONE BROTH DIET) | BELLY INCHES LOST: 1

Fran says, "I love that you can do a short-term plan like this and see results!" She'd already lost more than forty pounds on my original Bone Broth Diet, but she'd plateaued, and this diet empowered her to quickly take off some of those last stubborn pounds. She adds that before the Bone Broth Diet and the 10-Day Belly Slimdown, "No other weight-loss program has worked for me."

Fran, who's a savvy budgeter, found the bones for her broth at a farmer's market. She also bought an Instant Pot to make her broth, reusing the bones so she could get double the amount of broth from each batch of bones.

After the ten days, Fran says, her belly felt flatter. She adds, "My belly felt healthier and cleaner. I didn't have heartburn, I didn't have any discomfort in my belly, I didn't have constipation." In addition, she slept better during her diet, and she says, "I think my skin looks a little brighter." She was also delighted to discover that she had plenty of energy during the diet to keep up with her yoga and walking.

ter's princess doll down the toilet. Taking a quick break to write a "gratitude" list can lower your stress by helping you put things in perspective.

This is a simple technique you can do anywhere. Simply list (mentally or on paper) ten people or things for which you're grateful; these can be anything from your best friend to a fab new pair of shoes you just found on sale. Because it's hard to be stressed and grateful at the same time, this simple activity can help you chill out fast.

All these strategies will help you get control over your stress, as long as you make them a habit. So make time for at least one de-stressor *every single day*. No matter how wild life gets, find a little time to meditate, do Tai Chi, write in your journal, watch a silly YouTube video, or make a "gratitude" list. Remember: You're doing it for your belly!

A Quick Word About Diet Saboteurs

There's still another way you can reduce your stress during this diet—and that's by minimizing the damage done by people I call *diet saboteurs.*

We all know these people. They're our friends, our partners, our coworkers, and even our moms . . . and for some reason, they're out to thwart us every time we diet. Over two decades, I've seen far too many diets derailed by people like these.

I don't want you to let these people stand in your way—not even your mom. This diet is hard work, and to succeed, you need to stay strong. You also need your peeps to be on your side, not secretly wishing for you to fail. Each time they try to sabotage you, it increases your stress and makes it harder for you to reach your goal.

So how can you keep saboteurs from getting in your way? Your best defense is to recognize sabotage when it's happening. Here are the forms it's likely to take and how to deal with each one:

The guilt trip: "What do you mean, you can't come to Sunday dinner? I guess our family traditions aren't important to you anymore."
One great response to this is to guilt the person right back. So in a firm but pleasant tone of voice, say something along the lines

of, "They'll always be important, Mom. But for the next ten days, it's even more important for me to get rid of this unhealthy fat that's putting me at higher risk for diabetes and cancer, don't you think?"

The just-one-bite line: "C'mon, you've earned it!"
When you hear this line, just smile and say, "When my ten days are up, then I will have earned it—check back with me then."

The outright sabotage: "I know you're dieting, but I couldn't resist bringing you chocolates, because I know you love them."
When someone pulls this stunt, think about the real message behind the act. There's a good chance that the person is actually thinking (possibly subconsciously), "If you lose that belly fat, you're going to look really hot—and that could change our relationship."

As a result, he or she may feel threatened. And what's the easiest way to address that threat? By tempting you to cheat.

Now, this doesn't make the diet saboteur a bad person. Nearly anyone can feel a little threatened when a friend or partner makes a lifestyle change. (Admit it: Wouldn't you feel a bit insecure if your best friend suddenly got hotter, sexier, and a dress size smaller? Don't lie to me. You know you would.)

So don't get mad. Simply stand your ground politely, hand back the treats, and say, "I really appreciate the thought, but I'll need to pass right now."

The "Why change?" line: "Just learn to love your body as it is."
There's a big nugget of truth in this one, because you should respect your body rather than believing that you need to look like a model or a movie star to be attractive. However, that doesn't mean that you should accept having a big belly that puts you at risk for diabetes, heart disease, or even cancer.

My favorite reply to the "Why change?" line is, "I'm happy being me, but I want to be *the best me* I can be." Who can argue with that?

HOW MEDITATION HELPS YOU BLAST BELLY FAT

EMILY FLETCHER, FOUNDER, ZIVA MEDITATION

Meditation is becoming all the rage. Even if you aren't doing it yet, you probably know that it can improve the health of your brain. But you may not have heard that meditation can actually help you lose weight and reduce belly fat.

THE #1 MISCONCEPTION ABOUT MEDITATION

Before we dive into the science of why meditation can slim your belly, let's cover the number one most common misconception about meditation. When I tell people I am a meditation teacher, one of the first things out of their mouths is, "I would love to meditate. I have tried, **but I can't stop my mind from thinking.** My brain is just too crazy."

I'm not sure who keeps telling everyone that to meditate, you have to clear your mind, but I wish I could find this person and teach him or her to meditate.

If you have ever felt frustrated during meditation because you couldn't stop thinking about your taxes, your ex, or what snack you will make as soon as you finish this meditation thing, listen up: The mind thinks involuntarily, just like the heart beats involuntarily.

That's right: Your mind is doing its thing automatically, just like your liver, your nails, and your heart. You can't give your heart a command to stop beating. Similarly, you can't give your brain a command to be silent. Yet this is the criterion by which most people judge themselves when it comes to meditation.

The great news is that you are not a meditation failure, even if you were making very elaborate to-do lists during your last "failed" meditation attempt.

THE MEDITATION/WEIGHT CONNECTION

Once you find a meditation tool that works for you and develop a daily habit of meditation, your body starts to let go of a lifetime of accumulated stress. This also helps it to let go of a lifetime of accumulated weight.

When the body is stressed—whether the stress is emotional, physical, or due to past trauma—the brain and body flood with adrenaline and cortisol. These chemicals are acidic in nature and can cause an increase in inflammation. Additionally, cortisol is the chemical of survival. It tells the body to do everything it can to stay alive, which includes storing fat for the winter or an emergency.

Meditation is the most powerful stress-relieving tool we have. So it stands to reason that if you have a daily meditation practice, you will have less cortisol and adrenaline in your body, which can reduce inflammation and actually cue the body to release the "emergency" fat it was holding on to.

This is big, because emotional obesity affects as many as 80% of people with extra weight. Meditation can help decrease binge eating and emotional eating, leading to weight loss. It does this by giving you access to your bliss and fulfilment in the only place they exist, inside of you. Once your body starts to realize that it has access to this internal fulfillment on a repeatable and self-sufficient basis, it stops looking for happiness externally. The old story of "If I just have one more glass of wine or one last bite of ice cream . . . then I will be happy" starts to fade away. Meditation also helps the body release stored stress that can trigger this behavior.

While meditation is a deeply restful practice that helps get rid of the adrenaline and cortisol that can lead to fat storage, and specifically belly fat, mindfulness—which is more of a waking state practice—closes the feedback loop between the brain and the body. Any sensation your body gives you is trying to communicate something. If you don't listen, the sensations will get louder and louder. This can happen with cravings, physical pain, or emotions. Mindfulness gives you a way to check in with your body. It encourages you to listen for the subtle cues when the body whispers, which keeps it from having to yell.

MEDITATION AND MINDFULNESS IN ACTION

Researchers at the University of California at San Francisco have studied whether meditation and eating mindfully can reduce belly fat, even without reducing total body weight. The researchers also wanted to determine if these techniques could reduce emotional eating.

The researchers found that emotional eating decreased in people who meditated and ate mindfully. Overall, participants in the study reported less anxiety, less desire to eat as a reaction to emotions, and more awareness of body sensations. Loss of belly fat also occurred, even without a change in body weight.

MY EXPERIENCE

Meditation has transformed my personal relationship with food from a reward/punishment system into a healthy love affair. I now see food as a way to fuel and nourish my body and creativity. I no longer punish myself for or with it. Meditation has allowed me to eat more intuitively, because I am no longer addicted to food. I am not reaching to food as a way to fill myself up emotionally, which allows me to trust my instincts about what my body is asking for and when.

WHERE CAN YOU START?

Meditation is like any other skill. It takes a bit of training and, ideally, a technique that is designed for you. If you are ready to incorporate mindfulness and meditation into your daily health habits, check out our online training at zivameditation.com or find a teacher in your hometown who resonates with you.

Finally, keep diet saboteurs at bay by surrounding yourself with that inner circle of true friends I talked about earlier. Spend as much time as you can with peeps who'll cheer you on and be delighted for you when you show off your new, sexy body (even if they *are* a little jealous). Rather than stressing you out and making you feel like quitting, people like this will inspire you to stay the course.

By the way, if you're not sure how to talk with friends and family about your diet, try out my dinner party pitch. Here's how it goes:

> I love being healthy, feeling really energized, and losing my belly fat. Eating real, unprocessed foods does this for me.
>
> The concept is simple, really. It's just eating foods that my body metabolizes and digests best, so I can function better. Eating real, clean foods is helping me trim my waist, it's making my skin look better, and it's giving me tons of energy.

This diet is easier than you think, and the food tastes fantastic. For me, it's a no-brainer. I love the food, I love the way I look, and I love the way I feel.

You know what happens when I say this? Almost invariably, four or five people start asking me questions . . . and then they decide to go on the diet, too!

11

FLUSH OUT FAT WITH MY 10-DAY BELLY SLIMDOWN DETOX

Okay, don't hate me for this. I know I just told you to lower your stress levels, and now I'm going to drop a big fat stress bomb on you. (But read on, and I promise to de-stress you shortly!)

The bad news is that it's a dirty world out there, and every day you're bombarded with thousands of nasty chemicals—in your food, your water, your air, your household cleansers, and even your makeup. These chemicals can make you sick and fat, and there's no way to avoid all of them.

In fact, you're probably loaded with them right now. One study tested nine people—none of them working with chemicals on the job—and found 167 chemicals, pollutants, and pesticides in their blood and urine.[1]

The toxins in your body do very bad stuff. They cause inflammation, they slow your metabolism, and they pack on tons of that ugly, dangerous belly fat. Here's a quick sampling of the research showing how toxins can make your belly bigger:

- A long-term epidemiological study found a significant link between exposure to endocrine-disrupting chemicals such as bisphenol-A (BPA) and both obesity and type 2 diabetes.[2]

- Using data from the 1999–2002 U.S. National Health and Nutrition Examination Survey, researchers found a strong correlation between insulin resistance (one of the biggest causes of belly fat) and serum concentrations of persistent organic pollutants, especially for organochlorine compounds.[3]

- Researchers at Duke University recently exposed rats to high levels of air pollutants. After nineteen days, exposed male rats were 18% heavier than control rats breathing clean air, while female rats were 10% heavier.[4]

And BPA, organochlorine pesticides, and air pollutants are just some of the toxins identified as *obesogenic*—that is, they make you fat. There are many others, including—to name a few—cigarette smoke, flame retardants, organotins (tin-based chemicals used in industry and agriculture), and perfluorooctanoic acid (used in nonstick cookware).

Worse yet, research into obesogens is in its infancy. Researchers only began studying this issue a little more than a decade ago, so there undoubtedly are many, many more common toxins contributing to our epidemic of obesity.

I'm not going to lie to you: This is scary stuff.

However, I'm not here to scare you; I'm here to *empower* you. And the good news is that you're not just going to sit back and take it; you're going to fight back against these toxins.

In this chapter, you'll find out how to clean your body inside and out as it's never been cleaned before. As a result, you're going to be healthier, more energized, *and* slimmer.

My Three-Part 10-Day Belly Slimdown Detox

There are three steps to my 10-Day Belly Slimdown Detox. When you do my diet, you'll already be putting the first two steps into motion. Here they are:

- You'll load your body with foods that scrub it clean internally, revving up your detoxification machinery and transforming your cellular matrix—the fluid that your cells swim in—from sludgy to sparkling.

- You'll turn your skin into a strong barrier against toxins by eating cell-strengthening fats, loads of collagen, and foods rich in skin-healing nutrients—for instance, lauric acid, hyaluronic acid, and vitamin C.

Now let's talk about the third phase of my plan: making your personal world cleaner and safer, *one easy swap at a time.*

My Simple Trick: The Swap-a-Week Plan

I know it's easy to freak out when you think about all the places that toxins are hiding.

They're in your lipstick. Your face creams. Your shampoos. Your disinfectant wipes, weed killers, detergents, fabric softeners, and hair dye. Your plastic food-storage containers and plastic water bottles. They're even in your soap.

Think too hard about all this, and you may want to hide in bed all day. Of course, you may even be afraid to stay there, because who knows what chemicals are lurking in the laundry detergent and fabric softener you used when you washed your sheets?

But don't panic, because I have good news. You don't need to aim for a toxin-free body, which is an impossible goal. Instead, you can aim for a *doable* goal: reducing your overall *body burden* of toxins week by week.

Right now, your body may be overwhelmed with its heavy load of toxic "trash." But with each toxic chemical you remove, it'll get easier for your body's own detoxification systems to keep your insides clean and sparkly.

So here's what I want you to do. I call it my swap-a-week plan. It's practical, it's as inexpensive as going "clean" can be, and it'll slash your body burden of toxins. Here's how it works.

If you're like me, you run out of something each week—whether it's blush, dishwashing liquid, hair conditioner, or sunscreen. So at the end of each week, simply pick one "unclean" product that you ran out of, and swap it out for a "green" one. From that point on, continue to buy the nontoxic brand.

Follow this simple plan, and your body burden of toxins will drop every single week. Within months, that can add up to hundreds of chemicals that won't be winding up in your body—and within a year, it may add up to thousands. How's that for awesome?

I know that nontoxic products are more expensive than the "dirty" brands, and you don't have money to burn. So when you make your swaps, look for ways to cut your costs. For instance:

- Shop the sales. If you're willing to be flexible and try a variety of brands, you're likely to find some deep discounts.

- Use long-lasting bar soaps, or dilute liquid soaps with water so you can get more mileage from them.

- Swap out store-bought for homemade. For instance, use coconut oil or olive oil as a skin cream. Try old-fashioned household cleaners—vinegar, salt, and baking soda. And nuke those weeds with gardening vinegar (which is stronger than regular vinegar), or eliminate them the old-fashioned way: pull them by hand. Check out Pinterest for more great do-it-yourself ideas for cosmetics, cleansers, and yard-care products.

- Save a ton by buying products in bulk or using Amazon's Subscribe & Save feature.

SWAP-A-WEEK LIST

Here's a handy checklist you can use to track your prog-ress in detoxifying your world. The more of these you check off, the healthier you'll be—and the easier it'll be to keep that belly fat off forever!

MAKEUP

- ☐ Blush
- ☐ Eyeliner
- ☐ Eye shadow
- ☐ Foundation
- ☐ Lip balm
- ☐ Lipstick
- ☐ Mascara
- ☐ Nail polish
- ☐ Nail polish remover

HAIR, DENTAL, AND SKIN-CARE PRODUCTS

- ☐ Bath bombs
- ☐ Body butter
- ☐ Body wash
- ☐ Deodorant
- ☐ Face masks
- ☐ Face powder
- ☐ Hair conditioner
- ☐ Hair dye
- ☐ Hair mousse
- ☐ Hairspray
- ☐ Hair gel
- ☐ Moisturizers
- ☐ Mouthwash
- ☐ Perfume
- ☐ Shampoo
- ☐ Skin lotion
- ☐ Soap
- ☐ Suntan lotion
- ☐ Tanning oil
- ☐ Toothpaste
- ☐ Wrinkle cream

CLEANERS

- ☐ Air fresheners
- ☐ Bathroom cleaners
- ☐ Carpet shampoo
- ☐ Cleaning wipes
- ☐ Dishwasher pods or liquid
- ☐ Fabric softener
- ☐ Floor-care products
- ☐ Furniture polish
- ☐ Glass cleaner
- ☐ Laundry detergent
- ☐ Oven cleaner
- ☐ Toilet bowl cleaner

HOME AND YARD ITEMS

- ☐ Bug killers
- ☐ Insect repellants
- ☐ Weed killers

VISCERAL FAT AND ENVIRONMENTAL TOXINS

ANN SHIPPY, MD, FUNCTIONAL MEDICINE PHYSICIAN

Founder, Toxicity Matters® Foundation

Author of *Shippy Paleo Essentials* and *Mold Toxicity Workbook: Assess Your Environment & Create a Recovery Plan*

When I see patients in my office who are concerned about gaining belly fat and not being able to lose it, I let them know that this problem usually isn't just due to an imbalance of "calories in and calories out." One of the most common causes of resistant belly fat is *environmental toxin overload*.

As a physician practicing functional medicine, I get to run tests that most physicians don't even know about. Some of the tests I run when I suspect that toxicity is contributing to a patient's health problems are genetic tests examining the detoxification pathways (how our bodies get rid of things), tests measuring levels of toxins, and tests measuring levels of nutrients that run our physiology.

Our bodies are intelligent systems that are usually great at defending against natural threats and infections, but they often struggle with the removal of man-made threats such as chemicals from plastics, pesticides, cleaners, and furnishings. Human beings and elements of nature have coexisted for thousands of years, but man-made toxins have been around for less than a hundred years and are rapidly increasing annually. We have not evolved fast enough to combat these foreign, unnatural substances.

Complex chemical environments are, unfortunately, a normal part of our daily lives. Most of us can tolerate this influx of chemicals until our bodies get overwhelmed, leading to symptoms including weight gain, fatigue, chronic disease states such as diabetes, cancer, autoimmunity, heart disease, and more.[5, 6, 7, 8]

When overwhelmed, the adipose cells (a.k.a. "fat cells") become the "jail cells" that hold on to the chemicals and threats that the body is unable to eliminate. When the toxins are "incarcerated," they pose little threat to our vital organs and tissues, but they affect the adipose cells by causing them to expand and create new cells. The adipose cells increase in size but also require more "guards" in the form of macrophages and other immune-system cells.

These "guards" worsen the situation by secreting substances that lead to insulin resistance of the adipocytes.[9] Insulin resistance is associated with diabetes and weight gain.

Paula Baillie-Hamilton first proposed a link between environmental toxins and belly fat and metabolic disorders in 2002, when she noted rates of obesity increased in proportion to the increased production of synthetic chemicals. This eventually led to the "Environmental Obesogen Hypothesis," proposed by Grun and Blumberg in 2006, which led to many epidemiological studies and subsequent animal studies on the effects of chemicals on the body.[10, 11]

Environmental toxins that affect our health fall within the following seven categories:

- Highly fluorinated chemicals found in oil-, stain- and water-repellant products (e.g., GORE-TEX, nonstick cookware), food packaging, cosmetics, and more.

- Antimicrobial agents found in cleaning and personal-care products, clothing, exercise mats, and more.

- Flame retardants found in furniture, building materials, car seats, mattresses, building insulation, and more.

- Endocrine Disrupting Chemicals (EDCs), including bisphenols and phthalates, found in plastics (such as food storage containers), shower curtains, air fresheners, toys, and skin- and hair-care products.

- Solvents found in products such as cosmetics, dry cleaning agents, household cleaners, nail polish remover, and more.

- Metals such as mercury, arsenic, cadmium, and lead found in food, cookware, vaccines, makeup, dental fillings, jewelry, contaminated water, and more.

- Toxic mold that can be found in buildings and foods.

The most dangerous of these environmental pollutants are the persistent organic pollutants (a.k.a. POPs), which fall within the endocrine-disrupting chemicals category. Just as their name implies, they *persist* in the environment and in the human body—that is, they are difficult to remove. Why are they so harmful? The short answer is that the body has difficulty metabolizing or eliminating them.[12]

In 2001, the United Nations formed the Stockholm Convention to address the production and use of POPs. According to this treaty, countries that sign it agree to stop the production and use of the twelve worst POPs. The United States is not yet a contributing party on this treaty, but there has been a drop in the use of particular harmful substances.[13, 14]

Why do these chemicals collect in fat cells? The answer lies in the molecular structure of environmental toxins. Many are what we would call *lipophilic*, which means they are attracted to fat. In the body, the highest concentration of fat cells is in our abdomen (around our organs), in breast milk, and in the brain. Some chemicals, such as POPs, have a molecule that enhances their attraction to fat cells.[15, 16]

SUMMARY

"Incarcerating" environmental toxins in adipose tissue is a smart way our body protects us from unnatural and potentially harmful substances, but we obviously get frustrated by this system, because it eventually leads to belly fat, premature aging, and fatigue.

We can diminish the effects of environmental toxins by learning the sources of toxins, decreasing our exposure to them, and optimizing the removal of toxins via our gut and our skin. The best things to start eliminating from your life are sources of POPs and EDCs. This initially takes sacrifice, particularly for women (like it or not, we are often "addicted" to the cosmetics, skin-care products, interior decorating items, and clothing lines that are contributing to the toxin burden!). Here are some first steps to reduce your exposure to environmental toxins:

- **Fatty animal meats (particularly factory-farmed beef, poultry, and pork):** Replace with pasture-raised meats and wild-caught seafood.

- **Animal milk:** Replace with organic nut milks, ideally in glass containers.

- **Plastics involved in food packaging:** Replace with home-prepared meals, and store leftovers in glass containers; avoid water and beverages sold in plastic bottles.

- **Pesticides and herbicides (the worst is glyphosate, found in Roundup—don't use this in your yard!):** Replace with chemical-free weed killers, and choose organic produce (with a focus on the Environmental Working Group's list of the "Clean 15").

- **Skin-care products (even those from "natural" markets):** Replace with products that are rated a 1 through 3 according to the Environmental Working Group (use the phone app "Healthy Living" or "Think Dirty"); let your nails go natural.

- **Deodorant:** Eliminate brands with aluminum.

- **Furniture:** Avoid flame retardants and stain protection.

- **Air fresheners:** Don't use them!

- **Cleaners:** Swap toxic brands for clean ones.

- **Water:** Filter it.

- **Other toxins:** Eat 1 cup of organic cruciferous veggies each day to support your detoxification pathways.

With some savvy shopping and a little creativity, you can replace just about any product with a nontoxic version. And you can do it in a budget-friendly way by swapping out a single product at a time.

Here's a caution, however. Not every product that claims to be nontoxic truly is, so don't rely on advertising claims. Instead, get the facts before you buy.

Luckily, there's an easy way to do this. When you're searching for healthy products, check out the Environmental Working Group's Skin Deep database for info on cosmetics, lotions, soaps, and other skin-care products (ewg.org/skindeep) and their Guide to Healthy

Cleaning for info on household cleaning products (ewg.org/guides/cleaners).

Want to clean up your world even more? Here are two more smart swaps you can make:

- Swap out plastic containers for glass ones. Research shows that even BPA-free plastic containers leach synthetic estrogens that can put weight on you. In fact, some may be even *worse* for your waistline than containers that contain BPA.[17]

- Swap out nonstick pans for greener versions lined with ceramic.

Both these swaps are easy to make and will reduce your body burden of obesogens.

One Swap That Can't Wait: Dirty Water for Clean!

While my swap-a-week strategy will lower your body burden of toxins over time, there's one change I want you to make right now—and that's to purify your water. No matter how tight your budget is, this one can't wait.

Stop and think for a minute about how much water you use every day. You shower in it. You drink glasses of it each day. You make tea and coffee with it, wash your dishes in it, and add it to your food. That's a lot of water—and if you're getting it right from the tap, that water is disgusting. Bleah. Ick. Yuck.

You're probably aware of the tragedy in Flint, Michigan, where the tap water turned out to be heavily polluted with lead. But while the danger in Flint made headlines, I have bad news: *No matter where you live*, your tap water is toxic. For instance:

- The water in thirty-three U.S. states is contaminated with chemicals called PFASs, which are linked to obesity and cancer.[18]

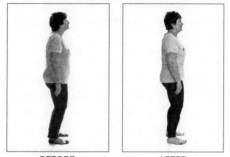
- Tap water in forty-two states is contaminated with 141 unregulated chemicals. (If you want to scare yourself silly, go to the Environmental Working Group's Natural Drinking Water Database and see what's in your local water.)[19]

- Dozens of U.S. cities are accused of "cheating" in an attempt to conceal problems with lead pollution in their tap water.[20]

Many toxins that wind up in your water—from pesticide residues to hormones to chemicals used in pipes to the herbicide atrazine—are known obesogens. In one recent study, the Environmental Working Group identified forty-five chemicals in tap water that are linked to hormonal disruption (a key cause of belly-fat gain).[21]

The good news is that it isn't all that expensive to clean up your water. Even if you're practically broke, you can save your pennies to buy a water filtration pitcher or a faucet filter. Point-of-use filters for your showers are also inexpensive. If you have some extra cash on

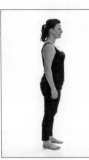
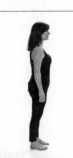

BEFORE   AFTER

JENNA KRUMLAUF

WEIGHT LOST: 12 POUNDS | BELLY INCHES LOST: 3.1

Jenna is a member of my own staff, but even after witnessing many of my weight-loss transformations, she was a little nervous about trying the diet. (I confess that I had to twist her arm a little.) Now, however, she's all smiles, because she lost more than *three inches* of belly fat in just ten days.

Her take on the diet? "Brace yourself. It's hard, but the quick benefits when you're 100% compliant are *incredible.*"

hand, a whole-house filtration system will do the job beautifully. The Environmental Working Group has an online Water Filter Guide to help you make smart choices that suit your budget.

So suck it up and buy the best water purifier you can afford. It may set you back a few bucks for a pitcher—or a few hundred dollars, if you go for a filtration system—but you and a slim belly are worth it. And seriously . . . do you *really* want hormones in your tea or herbicides in your minestrone?

Bottom Line: Clean Food, Clean Home, and Clean Water = Clean, Beautiful, Skinny You!

I know I'm asking a lot of you in this chapter. Even if you follow my simple swap-a-week plan, replacing toxic products with nontoxic ones takes work. What's more, it can be hard to kiss your favorites goodbye.

I confess that I wanted to cry a little when I swapped out the lipstick I'd adored for years—parabens, synthetic colors, and all—for a brand that wasn't going to kill me. It took me a while to convince myself that a lipstick that literally was "to die for" was *not* a good thing!

So, yes . . . I feel your pain. And I also feel the pain in your wallet, because going clean will make a slightly bigger dent in your paycheck.

But believe me, there's a big payoff. Every toxin you get out of your body will make you younger-looking, more energetic, and healthier—and as the science shows, lowering your body burden of toxins will also help keep those extra inches off your belly. So don't hesitate . . . start cleaning up your act!

And speaking of keeping those extra inches off, it's time for me to share my biggest secret for nuking that muffin top for good, *without* starving or sacrificing your favorite foods. It's my Slim Belly Forever plan, and it's going to banish your belly blues permanently. Get ready to say goodbye to constant yo-yo dieting and hello to food freedom.

PART IV

KISS YOUR BELLY FAT GOODBYE FOREVER!

Now that you have a beautiful belly, I'm going to tell you how to keep it that way. It's all about the magic of my Slim Belly Forever plan.

12

MY SLIM BELLY FOREVER PLAN

I f you've lost all the weight you want to lose, congratulations—you did it! And if you've jump-started your weight loss but still have more pounds to lose, you can switch now to my Bone Broth Diet. It's a less rigorous, long-term diet that'll strip the rest of those pounds off your belly.

Either way, when you get that beautiful belly you desire, you're going to feel lots of emotions. You're going to feel proud, relieved, sexy, and happy.

But you know what else you may feel?

A little scared.

Why? Because you've succeeded temporarily at diets before, but then you've put the weight right back on. Over and over and over again.

But guess what: I'm not going to let that happen.

My goal is for you to eat *fearlessly* for the rest of your life. I want you to enjoy all the foods you love, while keeping your belly slim for life.

And I know just how you'll do this: with my Slim Belly Forever plan. On this plan, *no* foods will be taboo. You'll be able to eat *anything you want* for 20% of your meals. You can have pancakes for breakfast on Sunday or pizza for dinner on Wednesday. And you'll do it without gaining weight. Sound too good to be true? Here's how it works.

Why the Slim Belly Forever Plan Is Magic

How can you get away with "cheating" 20% of the time? Simple. For the other 80% of your meals, you'll follow a healthy maintenance diet. This "80/20" style of eating is the basis of my Slim Belly Forever plan, and it's my secret for lifelong, sustained weight loss.

Each of your "80%" meals will include a protein, a serving of healthy fat, and as many non-starchy vegetables as you want. You can also include a little fruit, as well as a starchy veggie such as beets, carrots, or butternut squash if you need an extra shot of energy.

Here's how to build a perfect plate for each "80%" meal:

A PERFECT PLATE FOR YOUR SLIM BELLY FOREVER PLAN—*AFTER* YOU LOSE THE BELLY FAT!

PROTEIN PORTIONS

A serving of meat, fish, or poultry should be about the size and thickness of your palm. A serving of eggs is as many as you can hold in your hand (that's two or three for women, three or four for men). A serving of egg whites alone is double the serving for whole eggs. Each meal should include a serving of protein.

Note: Don't skimp on your protein! In fact, if you desire, you can increase your protein portion by half. The more we're learning about protein, the more we're finding that people—especially women—need plenty of it to stay young, strong, and healthy.

NON-STARCHY VEGETABLE PORTIONS

A serving of non-starchy vegetables should be at least the size of a softball. These are fabulous for you, so, if possible, fill your plate with at least two or three softballs' worth!

STARCHY VEGETABLE PORTIONS

A serving of starchy vegetables (such as sweet potato, jicama, kohl-rabi, or winter squash) should be about the size of a baseball for women and the size of a softball for men.

FRUIT PORTIONS

A serving of fruit is half an individual piece (half an apple, half an orange) or a tennis ball–size serving of berries, grapes, or tropical fruits. That's a closed handful, or about 1/2 cup, if they're diced. Eat no more than two servings of fruit per day, and break them up across meals and snacks to distribute your sugar intake.

FAT PORTIONS

A serving of oil or clarified butter is 1 tablespoon.

A serving of nuts, seeds, coconut flakes, or olives is about 1 closed handful.

A serving of nut butter is 1 tablespoon.

A serving of avocado is 1/4 to 1/2 an avocado.

A serving of coconut milk is 8 ounces, or 1/3 to 1/2 a can.

A serving of chia seeds is 4 teaspoons.

A serving of flaxseed is 2 tablespoons.

A serving of hemp seeds is 2 tablespoons.

When you eat this way 80% of the time, you'll build up enough good-food "credits" so that your indulgences won't do you any damage. As I like to say, you'll get 100% of the results for only 80% of the work.

Psychologically, this is a really big deal, because you'll never need to say, "I can't." One of the fastest ways to put weight back on your belly is to tell yourself that you can *never* have a food you enjoy—

whether it's ice cream, pizza, or macaroni and cheese. That's a guarantee that you'll crave it and that you'll gorge on it at some point.

So again: *No food is completely off-limits* on the Slim Belly Forever plan. Never say never. However, the closer you stick to a healthy template, the healthier you will be. So if you're battling a chronic health problem—for instance, psoriasis, irritable bowel syndrome, or an autoimmune condition—you may want to aim for 90/10 instead.

Also, as you switch to the 80/20 diet, be cautious about restarting two food groups in particular: dairy and grains. Contrary to popular belief, you don't need either one of these food groups in your diet. You can get plenty of calcium from nondairy foods such as salmon and leafy greens, and all the nutrients in grains are available from vegetables, proteins, and healthy fats.

Trust me: Your life will be better if you minimize dairy and grains in your diet or even kiss them goodbye. Here's why:

- Dairy is one of the biggest culprits behind bloating and gas. In addition, it can cause stomach cramps, loose bowel movements, and fatigue. Oh, and you know that embarrassing noise your GI tract makes during your morning stand-up meeting at work? Yeah, dairy can cause that, as well.

- Grains are inflammatory, so they're bad for your health. They age your inner belly, and in addition, they wreck your skin. And of course they're a major culprit in putting on belly fat! So giving up grains can do miracles when it comes to keeping your belly slim and clearing up acne, rosacea, and psoriasis.

I know that minimizing or eliminating grains can be tough. If you're not quite ready to let them go, at least reach for gluten-free grains such as quinoa, millet, buckwheat, aramanth, teff, and oats processed in a gluten-free facility. If you're a baker, try substituting almond or coconut flour for grain flours.

It goes without saying that there's one more food on my limit-or-ban list: sugar. It's fine to nibble on an occasional cookie or ice cream cone. However, the less sugar you eat, the less sugar you'll crave—and that will be good news for your belly *and* your health.

ARE YOU A SUGAR BURNER OR A FAT BURNER?

THE LINK BETWEEN SUGAR AND BELLY FAT

J. J. VIRGIN, CNS, BCHN, EP-C

Bestselling author of *JJ Virgin's Sugar Impact Diet: Drop 7 Hidden Sugars, Lose Up to 10 Pounds in Just 2 Weeks*

I often talk about how important it is to be a fat burner instead of a sugar burner, but what does that really mean? Instead of diving straight into the science, let's make this simple.

YOU KNOW YOU'RE A SUGAR BURNER IF . . .

. . . you rarely feel satisfied after a meal. Stuffed, maybe. Bloated and uncomfortable, yes. But ready to go another four to six hours without anything else to eat? No way!

. . . you snack regularly. You typically graze throughout the day, even when you've resolved to stop eating so much between meals. If you don't snack, you feel tired and moody.

. . . you struggle with belly fat. Even when you lose weight, it's from your arms and legs. You just can't seem to trim inches from your waist.

. . . you often get "hangry." You're no stranger to apologizing for being irritable because you were hungry. Your friends and family know that a bad attitude = hand you some food.

. . . you crave carbs and sugar. A meal isn't complete without potatoes, rolls, or pasta. Dessert is a must. And when you try to eat less sugar, you find yourself cranky and unable to focus.

If you recognize yourself in the descriptions above, you're probably a sugar burner. That means your primary source of fuel is glucose (blood sugar), which gives your body no reason to use your fat stores for fuel. Why should it, since you run on a steady supply of carbs?

Here's how it works: When you eat sugar or carbohydrates, your blood sugar rises. Then your pancreas releases insulin, a hormone that helps restore balance by pulling that excess sugar out of your bloodstream. The higher your blood sugar levels, the more insulin your body is forced to produce in order to return those levels to normal.

All that insulin comes with several major drawbacks, including blocking leptin production. Leptin is your appetite-control hormone. Without it, your brain never gets that signal that says you're full—that's why sugar burners are often hungry and overweight.[1]

THE DANGERS OF USING SUGAR FOR FUEL

It's a vicious cycle. Being a sugar burner means your body needs more insulin and hangs on to fat; in turn, high body fat makes you less responsive to insulin.[2] That insulin resistance causes its own set of problems, including increased risk of heart disease, type 2 diabetes, and inflammation.[3, 4] As a result, sugar burners often suffer from joint pain, headaches, skin trouble, and uncomfortable gut issues.[5, 6, 7]

Even when sugar burners lose weight, they seldom lose fat. And any time you lose *weight* without losing *waist*, you're actually making things worse! You're training your body to store your fat even more stubbornly.

The results can be miserable: Sugar burners often suffer from anxiety or depression, constant cravings, and obesity. In turn, being overweight and unhappy causes your body to produce more stress hormones such as cortisol. And guess what cortisol does? Raises your blood sugar and encourages your body to store more belly fat!

As if all that wasn't bad enough, with time, all those hormone spikes can cause symptoms ranging from high blood pressure to elevated cholesterol.[8, 9] It's time to get off the sugar roller coaster. . . .

WHAT IT MEANS TO BE A FAT BURNER

The goal is to be a fat burner instead. By eating fewer sugary carbs and more clean, lean protein, fiber, and healthy fats, you train your body to burn fat for fuel.

That's right—eat *more* fat! The old '80s myth that a low-fat diet leads to weight loss is well and truly busted.[10, 11, 12] In fact, it turns out that your body will only let go of extra pounds when it's sure you're not starving. The best way to send that message? Eat a balanced diet that includes healthy fats.[13, 14]

As a fat burner, your system still burns carbs as fuel first, and it will use the small amount of sugar you get from slow/low carbs—that is, foods that are low in carbs or have carbs that burn slowly—such as vegetables, quinoa, or legumes. Then your metabolism quickly turns to your fat stores for energy.

Because fat burns more slowly and steadily, fat burners can easily go four to six hours between meals and don't suffer from sugar or carb cravings.[15] They also lose fat easily and experience steadier energy.

MAKE SMART SWAPS

As you start cutting sugars out of your diet, watch out for sneaky sugars. That bran muffin and OJ you just had as part of your "healthy breakfast" actually contained around 70 grams of sugar! Trade your fancy frappe-style coffee for an unsweetened coconut milk latte, and you eliminate another 69 grams of sugar.

But the opportunities to become a fat burner don't end with your first meal of the day. That raspberry vinaigrette on your salad at lunch turned it into dessert by adding another 14 grams of sugar. (Try lemon juice and extra-virgin olive oil instead.)

At dinner, swap your side of whole wheat rigatoni for noodles made from lentil and quinoa flour (once you're on your Slim Belly Forever plan after the end of your diet). Not only do you lose the inflammatory gluten, you also gain 14 grams of filling, gut-healing fiber and 25 grams of fat-burning protein.

The options to lower your sugar impact are endless! And the more you eliminate syrupy-sweet foods, the more you'll reclaim your palate and truly start to taste your meals again.

All those symptoms you blamed on aging—stubborn belly fat, fatigue, bloating, joint pain—are actually symptoms of burning glucose for energy. If you're a sugar burner, it's not too late to stop the cycle of mood swings, brain fog, and weight gain. Your body *and* your loved ones will thank you!

If you can't give up sugar entirely, try to save sugary treats for very special occasions such as birthdays or holidays.

Also, if you really have a sweet tooth, give monk fruit sweetener a try. (It's typically in the same section as sugar in stores.) It has close

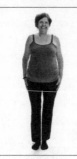 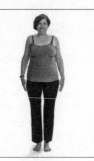

BEFORE   AFTER

DEBORAH PHILLIPS

WEIGHT LOST: 6.8 POUNDS | BELLY INCHES LOST: .75

Deborah says, "Overall I feel good, and I have not felt good for some time. I was gaining weight for no apparent reason, and now I have lost weight."

She adds that the plan is easy to follow and the results are incredible. "I have already recommended [it] to a friend," she says.

Deborah knew that she had food allergies or sensitivities, but she wasn't sure which foods were the culprits. Now she says, "With this program I feel like I have a fresh start and will be able to determine what I can and cannot eat as I add back some foods to my diet."

to zero calories, and it's safe for everyone, including diabetics. Monk fruit also contains antioxidants called *mogrosides*, and research on mice with induced diabetes found that mogrosides lower blood glucose, improve blood lipids, and reduce oxidative stress (damage to cells caused by free radicals).[16] I love monk fruit in shakes and smoothies, and it's heat stable, so you can bake with it, too.

Finally, put high-carb veggies such as sweet potatoes, carrots, and beets in their proper place. These are all terrific foods, but loading your plate with them will put that belly fat right back on you. Instead, think of these as *accents* for your plate, and on your "80%"

days, limit yourself to a spoonful or two—not an entire sweet potato or a cup of cooked carrots.

Also, think of these carb-y veggies as energy boosters. If you do an intense workout and you feel wobbly, add one of them to your next meal. But if you're having an easy day, substitute a non-starchy veggie instead.

Why I Want You to Stop Grazing

If you were a "grazer" before you started my 10-Day Belly Slim-down plan, you might be tempted to go back to your former habits once you're on the Slim Belly Forever plan. If so, I hope I can change your mind.

One of the most popular ideas in the fitness world today is that you should eat six or more small meals throughout the day. This sounds great, I know, because what's not to like about eating all day long? Well, here are six things I don't like about it, for starters:

- Eating all day long (especially if you're eating lots of carbs) keeps your insulin and leptin levels spiking all day long. The result: You develop both insulin resistance and leptin resistance, making you fat and hungry.

- When you eat all day long, your body gets into the habit of expecting frequent meals. As a result, you crave food even when you don't need it.

- Grazing can increase your risk of small-intestinal bacterial overgrowth, or SIBO. When you go for ninety minutes to two hours without eating, the muscles in your small intestine generate a "cleansing wave" that whooshes toxins out. When you snack all the time, you deactivate this wave. As a result, you create an unhealthy condition where gut bugs can overbreed.

- Grazing can promote constipation. After a large meal, you may feel the need to "go." That's because cues such as stomach distention tell your GI tract to make room for the food that's heading its way. When you eat small snacks all day, your gut may not get these cues—and as a result, your plumbing can get sluggish.

- Eating frequent meals that contain fruit or other carbs keeps your mouth in an acidic state. This, in turn, can lead to tooth decay.

- Grazing doesn't help you lose weight more easily. As the Salk Institute research I talked about in Chapter 1 shows, going for long periods *without* eating is the best way to take those pounds off—not snacking all day long.

If you're a grazer, the idea of cutting down to just a few meals a day may scare you. That's because you're worried that you'll get overwhelmingly hungry and wind up in the nearest pizza joint eating everything but the tablecloth.

However, here's the reality. Eating two or three low-carb meals a day will keep your blood sugar steady, rather than causing wild swings—and it's those swings that lead to cravings. And if you do get the urge to eat between meals, bone broth can satisfy your hunger fast, without any of the downsides of snacking.

So leave the grazing to the cows, and once you finish this diet, try to stick to a maximum of three meals each day (and maybe an occasional snack). You'll be less hungry, you'll have more control over your eating, and you'll keep your belly slim and happy.

What If the Pounds Start to Creep Back On?

Let's talk about something else: What if you get a little careless, and 80/20 turns into 70/30 or 60/40? If that happens, you'll probably start to notice your pants getting tight again.

In this case, don't panic, and don't kick yourself. We're all perfectly imperfect—and I'm right at the top of that list, so I'm the last person who's going to scold you. The solution is simple: Just do another ten days on the 10-Day Belly Slimdown—or, if you're in less of a hurry, follow the twenty-one-day plan I outline in *Dr. Kellyann's Bone Broth Diet*.

The biggest trick here is to nip this problem in the bud. It's easy to take off five pounds but not so easy to take off fifteen or twenty. So if you look in the mirror and see a little "pooch" reappearing, take action fast. Go right back on your diet plan, and you'll kiss that belly fat goodbye quickly.

Also, once you do take off those pounds, think about how you put them on. Were you OD'ing on chips, hitting the ice cream too hard, or indulging in too many wine coolers? When you identify the culprits that made those pounds sneak onto your belly, you can avoid falling prey to them in the future.

Five Tips for "Forever" Success

The Slim Belly Forever plan will keep your belly flat and sexy for life, as long as you do it right. Here are five keys to success:

AVOID "PORTION CREEP"

Over time, it's easy to let one serving of avocado turn into two or three, or to toss an extra serving of fruit into a protein shake. But those little cheats eventually add up to extra pounds on your belly. Follow my Perfect Plate template, and that won't happen.

One portion-control tip in particular: Be especially careful when you're snacking on nuts. These babies are delicious—and that's the problem. How often do you say, "I'm just going to have a handful," and then wind up sucking down a whole can of them? (Uh-huh. I thought so.) Remember that a serving of nuts is one closed handful, and stick to a maximum of one serving each day.

KEEP EATING THOSE HEALTHY FATS

Remember: *Eating healthy fats helps you lose fat.* Don't overdo it . . . but don't think that you're doing yourself any favors by going low-fat. Healthy fats keep your metabolism running on high so that belly fat doesn't sneak back on, and they also give you beautiful skin and hair. So add a dose of these fats to every meal.

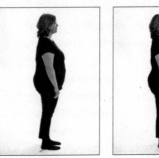

BEFORE   AFTER

MARIA HERBEL

WEIGHT LOST: 7.2 POUNDS | BELLY INCHES LOST: 1.5

Maria says her 10-Day Belly Slimdown was "the fastest weight loss I've ever had, with minimal pain as far as hunger and just feeling lousy. I think I had a little 'carb flu,' but every morning I woke up feeling more energetic."

Maria previously tried Atkins, Weight Watchers, and a score of other diets, with no success. This time, she says, "The bone broth really satisfied my urges to eat. I'd have a hard day at work, and during the day I'd think, 'I'll go get my bone broth.' And as soon as I'd start sipping on it—I don't know if I had a blood pressure drop or what happened, but I'd feel I calmed down."

One thing that tickled Maria was her husband telling her after the diet, "You know, you're my trophy wife."

"We've been married thirty-four years," she says, smiling, "and he hasn't said that in a while."

DRINK BONE BROTH AND ADD COLLAGEN TO YOUR DIET EVERY DAY

Staying in the bone broth and collagen habit even after your diet ends is a smart idea. It'll keep your gut healthy, reduce your inflammation, and fill you up so you're less tempted to put junk in your body. It'll also keep erasing your wrinkles—and who doesn't want that?

You can drink your broth straight, put it in soups and stews, or even add it to cocktails. (Really—it's delicious! I'll share some recipes in the next chapter.) As for collagen, you can add it to shakes and soups or enjoy a daily cup of my Collagen Coffee.

Also, if you have a slipup—for instance, if you eat *way* too much pizza and wind up bloated and three pounds heavier the next day— try doing a one-day bone broth mini-fast. This is easy (simply drink nothing but bone broth from the time you get up until the time you go to bed), and it'll erase the damage as if it never even happened.

KEEP MOVING . . . AND KEEP THAT STRESS UNDER CONTROL

When you're busy, I know it's tempting to backslide on exercising, journaling, or meditation. But these strategies matter *every bit* as much as what you put on your plate, so don't neglect them. No matter how hectic your life is, set aside some "you" time to work out or chill out. Remember, you're just as important as the people you're caring for.

ENJOY THE NEW YOU!

If you're used to hiding your belly fat and bloat, I'm betting that you have a closet full of baggy clothes. If that's the case, I want you to go out *right now* and buy yourself some sexy outfits. It's time to reap the rewards of your diet!

The more glances you get from hot guys or gals, and the more your friends admire (and envy) your beautiful belly, the more motivated you'll be to stick to your Slim Belly Forever plan. And that will guarantee that you'll keep that gorgeous belly.

So what are you waiting for? Go strut your stuff!

And while you're at it, celebrate with the yummy Slim Belly Forever recipes in the next chapter. These fun dishes will ease you right into a lifetime of belly-friendly eating.

RECIPES FOR YOUR SLIM BELLY FOREVER PLAN

O nce you reach your goal weight, you can let a little indulgence tiptoe back into your life. So let me introduce you to some of my favorite only-slightly-sinful treats.

These recipes are a teeny bit wicked because they include ingredients such as ancient grains, honey, and even a little vodka. But they won't do you a bit of harm, as long as you limit them to 20% of your meals.

So go ahead—treat yourself. Whip up some Lemon "Cheesecakes" with Berry Topping for a girls' night, enjoy my Chicken Enchiladas Verdes for dinner, or toast your diet success with a Skinny Moscow Mule. *Salud!*

BROTH WITH VEGGIES

PREP TIME: **35 MIN.** | YIELD: **4 SERVINGS**

Many thanks to my friend Karen Pickus, chef and food stylist at Good Morning America, *who developed this hearty, veggie-packed broth for the book.*

1 quart Chicken Bone Broth (page 96)

2 carrots, sliced $1/2$ inch thick

1 parsnip, peeled and sliced $1/2$ inch thick

$1/2$ yellow onion, diced small

1 large garlic clove, minced

$1/2$ teaspoon dried thyme

$1/2$ teaspoon ground turmeric

$3/4$ cup full-fat coconut milk

$1 1/2$ cups fresh baby spinach

In a large stockpot, bring the broth to a simmer over medium heat. Add the carrots, parsnip, onion, garlic, thyme, and turmeric. Simmer, uncovered, for 15 minutes, until the vegetables are tender. Add the coconut milk and spinach, stir, turn off the heat, and cover. Allow the spinach to wilt, 5 to 10 minutes.

Recipe courtesy Karen Pickus • Recipe written and developed by Karen Pickus

CHICKEN AND BEANS BOWL

PREP TIME: **40 MIN.** | YIELD: **1 SERVING**

Here's another treat from Good Morning America *chef and food stylist Karen Pickus. It's loaded with spices that will rev up your metabolism!*

CHICKEN

1 small skinless, boneless chicken breast (4 ounces), butterflied

1/8 teaspoon ground cumin

1 garlic clove, minced

1/8 teaspoon ground coriander

1/8 teaspoon chili powder

Salt and freshly ground black pepper

1 teaspoon olive oil

BEANS

1/2 cup cooked black beans

1/4 yellow onion, minced

1 garlic clove, minced

1/8 teaspoon ground cumin

Salt and freshly ground black pepper

1 cup kale leaves

1 cup arugula

Drizzle of olive oil

Juice of 1/4 lime

Make the chicken. In a medium bowl, combine the chicken with the spices. Drizzle the olive oil over top and stir to combine. Cover with plastic wrap and set aside.

Make the beans. Meanwhile, in a small pot, combine the black beans, onion, garlic, cumin, and salt and pepper to taste, and bring to a boil over high heat. Remove from the heat and cover to keep warm.

In a medium skillet, cook the seasoned chicken over medium-high heat for 3 to 4 minutes per side, until cooked through. Transfer to a plate.

To serve, place the black beans in a bowl and add the kale and arugula to the beans. Slice the grilled chicken and place it on top of the greens. Drizzle with olive oil and the lime juice.

Recipe courtesy Karen Pickus 2017 • Recipe developed and written by Karen Pickus 2017

BRUSCHETTA CHICKEN

PREP TIME: **15 MIN.** | COOK TIME: **20 MIN.** | YIELD: **4 SERVINGS**

CHICKEN

1 tablespoon avocado oil

4 boneless, skinless chicken breasts

1/2 teaspoon Celtic or pink Himalayan salt

1/2 teaspoon freshly ground black pepper

1/4 teaspoon garlic powder

1/2 teaspoon Italian seasoning

BRUSCHETTA TOPPING

6 Roma tomatoes, seeded and cut into 1/4-inch cubes

1/2 cup basil leaves, cut into fine ribbons

1 tablespoon olive oil

1 garlic clove, smashed

1/4 teaspoon Celtic or pink Himalayan salt

Freshly ground black pepper

1 to 2 teaspoons balsamic vinegar

Crushed red pepper, for serving

Make the chicken. In a large skillet, heat the oil over medium-high heat. Meanwhile, in a shallow dish, season the chicken with the salt, black pepper, garlic powder, and Italian seasoning.

Once the oil is hot, add the seasoned chicken to the pan and cook for 7 to 10 minutes per side, depending on the thickness of the chicken, until cooked through.

Make the bruschetta topping. While the chicken is cooking, put all the bruschetta topping ingredients in a large bowl and stir to combine.

To serve, arrange the chicken on a serving platter and top each piece with some bruschetta. Serve with the crushed red pepper.

NOTES: You can also make the bruschetta topping a few hours before preparing the chicken so the flavors can meld. Let the topping come to room temperature before spooning it onto the chicken. If you care to use cheese, you may grate any hard, aged cheese over the dish when serving.

CHICKEN ENCHILADAS VERDES

PREP TIME: **20 MIN.** | COOK TIME: **30 MIN.** | YIELD: **2 SERVINGS**

Coconut or avocado oil cooking spray

1 pound fresh tomatillos, or 2 (11-ounce) cans tomatillos, sugar-free, drained and rinsed

1 cup Chicken Bone Broth (page 96)

1/2 medium onion, roughly chopped

1 garlic clove, minced

1 tablespoon chopped fresh cilantro

1 serrano chile or jalapeño, roughly chopped

1/2 teaspoon Celtic or pink Himalayan salt (omit if using canned tomatillos)

1 to 2 teaspoons arrowroot powder, blended with 1 to 2 tablespoons water

4 Siete Foods grain-free tortillas (see Notes)

2 cups cooked and shredded chicken from Roast Chicken with Herbs and Lemon (page 135) or a rotisserie chicken

1 tablespoon plus 1 teaspoon nutritional yeast (optional)

Preheat the oven to 350°F. Spray a 9 x 9-inch baking pan with cooking spray.

In a blender or food processor, combine the tomatillos, broth, onion, garlic, cilantro, serrano, and salt and blend until smooth.

Transfer the sauce to a saucepan and bring it to a boil over medium heat. Reduce the heat to low and simmer for about 10 minutes.

Add the arrowroot mixture by the teaspoon, stirring until the sauce thickens. Remove from the heat and pour 1 cup of the sauce onto a rimmed plate. Set aside.

Spray a sauté pan with cooking spray. Set the pan over medium-high heat. When hot, add a tortilla and heat for about 15 seconds per side. They can also be heated in a plastic bag in the microwave in 5-second intervals.

Dip the warmed tortillas into the plated sauce one at a time. To each tortilla, add 1/2 cup cooked chicken and 1/4 cup of the sauce. Gently roll them up and set seam side down in the prepared baking pan. Pour the remaining sauce over the enchiladas, cover with foil, and bake for 20 to 25 minutes.

NOTES: If you are going to poach the chicken rather than use roasted chicken, 1 pound boneless breast, thigh, or a combination thereof is equal to about 2 cups.

For a "cheesy" flavor, sprinkle 1 teaspoon nutritional yeast over each enchilada before rolling.

Siete Foods grain-free tortillas and tortilla chips are available at sietefoods.com

CHOCOLATE ALMOND TRUFFLES

PREP TIME: **15 MIN.** | YIELD: **20 TO 24 PIECES**

1/2 cup pitted dates

1/4 cup raw cacao powder or unsweetened cocoa powder

1/4 cup almond butter

1/2 cup almonds, toasted and finely chopped

1/2 teaspoon instant espresso powder

1 teaspoon pure almond or vanilla extract

Stevia or monk fruit sweetener to equal about 1 tablespoon sugar (optional)

Pinch of salt

In a food processor, combine the dates, cacao, almond butter, 1/4 cup of the almonds, the espresso powder, almond extract, stevia, and salt and pulse until the mixture forms a sticky ball.

Roll into 20 to 24 individual balls, and roll in the remaining toasted almonds to coat. Serve immediately or store in the refrigerator until 15 minutes before serving.

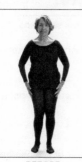
BEFORE

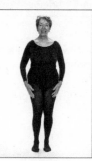
AFTER

ELIZABETH MCKENZIE

WEIGHT LOST: 7 POUNDS | BELLY INCHES LOST: 3

Elizabeth says she did the diet mainly to address immune-system issues. "It wasn't weight loss so much," she comments, "but that was a nice benefit!"

Elizabeth suffered from joint pain before starting the diet. She says, "I noticed the very first day that all my aches and pains were gone, which I thought was phenomenal." She credits this to cutting out high-carb foods such as bread—something she's been trying to do for years. With this diet, she says, "I was able to do it."

Overall, Elizabeth says that her health complaints were "about 75% gone" when she finished the diet. For instance, she says, "I used to have acid reflux, and I don't have it any-more."

I'm delighted to share Elizabeth's story because it brings up an important point. I know your main target right now is your belly fat—but when you cut unhealthy foods out of your diet, you get healthier *all over.* So in addition to trimming your belly, you'll enjoy everything from better skin and happier joints to freedom from acid reflux, gas, and bloating. That's pretty awesome, isn't it?

CILANTRO CHICKEN

PREP TIME: **15 MIN.** | COOK TIME: **15 MIN.** | YIELD: **4 SERVINGS**

4 boneless, skinless chicken breasts, pounded thin and cut into 2 or 3 pieces each

1/2 teaspoon onion powder

1/2 teaspoon Celtic or pink Himalayan salt

1/2 teaspoon white pepper

2 tablespoons pasture butter or ghee (page 147)

1 cup diced fresh Roma tomatoes

1/2 cup diced yellow onion

1 garlic clove, minced

1 1/2 cups Chicken Bone Broth (page 96)

1 teaspoon paprika

5 ounces canned full-fat coconut milk

1/2 cup roughly chopped fresh cilantro

1/2 jalapeño, minced (optional)

1/2 cup 1/2-inch cubes mango

1/3 cup canned black beans, drained and rinsed

In a shallow dish, season the chicken breasts with the onion powder, salt, and white pepper.

In a heavy skillet, melt 1 tablespoon of the butter over medium heat. Add the chicken and brown on each side, 3 to 4 minutes, until fully cooked. Transfer to a clean platter and keep warm.

In the same pan, melt the remaining 1 tablespoon butter and add the tomatoes, onion, and garlic. Cook for 5 minutes, until softened. Add the broth, paprika, and coconut milk and increase the heat to medium-high. Gently simmer to reduce the liquid by half.

Stir in the cilantro, jalapeño, mango, and black beans and simmer for a few more minutes. Remove from the heat and pour over the chicken.

NOTE: This is delicious over rice, cauliflower "rice" (see Note, page 158), or steamed spinach.

CITRUS SALAD WITH FENNEL

PREP TIME: **20 MIN.** | YIELD: **4 SERVINGS**

SALAD

6 cups arugula or a mix of arugula and frisée (curly endive)

1 fennel bulb, very thinly sliced

1 large or 2 small shallots, very thinly sliced

2 navel or Cara Cara oranges

1 pink grapefruit

1 blood orange (if they're in season; otherwise, use another type of orange)

1 avocado, sliced

Celtic or pink Himalayan salt

Freshly ground black pepper

ORANGE VINAIGRETTE

1/3 cup fresh orange juice

1 tablespoon champagne vinegar or white wine vinegar

1 tablespoon honey

1/3 cup avocado oil or olive oil

1 garlic clove, smashed

Pinch of cayenne pepper

Make the salad. In a large flat-bottomed bowl or platter, combine the arugula, fennel, and shallots.

Using a sharp knife, cut all the pith and peel from the oranges and grapefruit, then slice them into 1/4-inch-thick rounds. If the grapefruit rounds are very large, cut them in half. Add the oranges and grapefruit to the salad. Top with the avocado slices and season with salt and lots of freshly ground black pepper.

Make the dressing. In a small bowl or a jar with a tight-fitting lid, combine all the dressing ingredients. Whisk or shake to blend.

Drizzle the dressing over the salad (making sure to not include the garlic), toss, and serve. Refrigerate any remaining dressing.

NOTES: To quickly and easily get very thin slices of fennel and shallot, use a mandoline; otherwise, be sure your knife is very sharp.

Turn this salad into a meal by adding chilled cooked shrimp or chicken.

ASPARAGUS BUNDLES WRAPPED IN BACON

PREP TIME: **10 MIN.** | COOK TIME: **15 MIN.** | YIELD: **4 SERVINGS**

20 asparagus spears, about 5 inches long

4 strips center-cut nitrite-, nitrate-, and sugar-free bacon

Coconut or avocado oil cooking spray

Freshly ground black pepper

Zest and juice of 1/2 lemon

Preheat the oven to 400°F and place a rack in the center of the oven.

Wash the asparagus spears and arrange them in bundles of 5 on a cutting board. Wrap each bundle in the center with 1 strip of bacon to secure the bunch. If needed, use kitchen twine to tie each bundle. Place the bundles on a metal baking rack set inside of a rimmed baking sheet. Spray the asparagus with cooking spray and generously sprinkle with pepper.

Bake for 12 to 15 minutes, until the bacon is cooked. Remove from the oven and immediately drizzle with the lemon juice. Top with the lemon zest before serving.

CRAB AND AVOCADO SALAD

PREP TIME: **10 MIN.** | YIELD: **2 SERVINGS**

1 medium avocado, halved and pitted

Celtic or pink Himalayan salt

Squeeze of fresh lemon juice

4 to 6 ounces lump crabmeat

Green Goddess Dressing (page 153)

6 to 8 butter lettuce leaves

2 small tomatoes, cut into wedges

1/2 English cucumber, sliced into half-moons

1/2 small sweet onion, thinly sliced (optional)

Carefully spoon out the avocado halves. Place them on a plate, sprinkle them with salt, and squeeze the lemon juice over top.

In a medium bowl, combine the crabmeat with enough Green Goddess Dressing to moisten the crab.

Arrange the lettuce on two plates and top with the tomatoes, cucumber, and onion, if using. Divide the crab salad between the avocado halves and set them on top of the lettuce leaves. Serve any remaining dressing on the side.

NOTE: Green Goddess Dressing is also fabulous on a garden salad, served with fish or chicken, or used as a crudité dip.

LEMON "CHEESECAKES" WITH BERRY TOPPING

PREP TIME: **20 MIN. PLUS 4 TO 6 HOURS FOR FREEZING** | COOK TIME: **10 MIN.** | YIELD: **12 CUPCAKE-SIZE "CHEESECAKES"**

CRUST

- 3/4 cup sunflower seeds
- 1/4 cup pumpkin seeds
- 2 tablespoons unsweetened shredded coconut
- 1/2 cup pitted dates (about 12 small to medium), soaked in water for 20 minutes, then drained
- 1/4 teaspoon Celtic or pink Himalayan salt
- Coconut oil cooking spray

FILLING

- 3 cups raw, unsalted cashews, soaked in water overnight
- 3/4 cup fresh lemon juice
- 1 tablespoon lemon zest
- 1 1/2 teaspoons pure vanilla extract
- 3/4 cup coconut oil, melted
- 1/2 cup honey
- Pinch of Celtic or pink Himalayan salt

BERRY TOPPING (OPTIONAL)

- 2 cups berries (blueberries, blackberries, raspberries, strawberries, or mixed berries)
- 1 teaspoon honey or equivalent stevia or monk fruit sweetener
- 1/2 teaspoon pure vanilla extract

Make the crust. In a large, wide skillet, toast the sunflower seeds, pumpkin seeds, and coconut over low heat, stirring often, for about 15 minutes. Watch carefully, because it's easy to burn the mixture.

In a food processor, combine the toasted mixture, dates, and salt and pulse until just combined. The mixture should have a lot of texture.

Spray a muffin tin with cooking spray and pat about 1^1/$_2$ to 2 tablespoons of the crust mixture into the bottom of each cup. No need to press the crust up the sides.

Make the filling. When you are ready to make the filling, drain the cashews and pour half of them into a high-speed blender or food processor. Add the remaining ingredients and blend well. Add the remaining cashews and blend until the mixture is creamy and pourable. Pour into the prepared crusts and freeze for 4 to 6 hours, or until completely frozen.

Make the berry topping (if using). In a small saucepan, combine the berries and sweetener. Simmer over medium-low heat for 8 to 10 minutes, until the mixture becomes saucy but the fruit still retains some of its shape. Remove from the heat, add the vanilla, and set aside. Refrigerate when cool.

To serve, remove the cakes from the freezer and let them sit at room temperature for 5 to 10 minutes. Gently remove them from the pan with a small offset spatula and top with the berry topping, if using.

NOTES: These "cheesecakes" are equally delicious without the sauce. You can also top them with fresh fruit. If you are not serving them all at once, simply remove the number you want from the tin and refreeze the others.

MUSSELS WITH FENNEL AND SPICED PORK SAUSAGE

PREP TIME: **20 MIN.** | COOK TIME: **20 MIN.** | YIELD: **4 SERVINGS**

1/2 pound ground pastured pork

1 teaspoon chili powder

1/2 teaspoon garlic powder

1/2 teaspoon Celtic or pink Himalayan salt

1/2 teaspoon freshly ground black pepper, plus more to taste

Dash of cayenne pepper

2 tablespoons pastured butter or ghee (page 147)

1/2 fennel bulb, thinly sliced

3 garlic cloves, minced

1 small shallot, thinly sliced

1 pint cherry tomatoes, halved

2 cups Seafood (page 100) or Chicken (page 96) Bone Broth

2 pounds mussels, scrubbed and debearded

2 tablespoons roughly chopped Italian parsley, for serving

In a medium bowl, combine the pork, chili powder, garlic powder, salt, black pepper, and cayenne.

In a Dutch oven or stockpot, melt the butter over medium heat. Add the seasoned pork and, using a spatula, break it up into crumbles. Add the fennel, garlic, and shallot and cook for 3 to 4 minutes, until softened. Add the tomatoes and broth, reduce the heat to low, and simmer for 6 to 8 minutes, until the tomatoes begin to soften.

Add the mussels, cover, and cook, stirring occasionally, until the mussels open, 6 to 8 minutes. Discard any mussels that don't open. Serve the mussels in bowls topped with the broth and parsley.

"PUT THE LIME IN THE COCONUT" FAT BOMBS

PREP TIME: **10 MIN.** | YIELD: **ABOUT 20 FAT BOMBS**

1 cup coconut butter

1/4 cup coconut oil

Zest and juice of 2 small limes
(use a very fine grater to
avoid chunks)

1/2 teaspoon pure vanilla extract

Stevia or monk fruit sweetener
to equal 2 to 3 tablespoons
sugar

Pinch of Celtic or pink Himalayan
salt

Put the coconut butter and coconut oil in medium bowl and bring
them to room temperature so they are soft enough to easily combine.
If needed, you can warm them for a few seconds in the microwave.
Add the lime zest and juice, vanilla, sweetener, and salt and stir well
to evenly distribute the ingredients. Taste for sweetness and adjust
as needed.

Line a mini-muffin tin with paper liners and spoon about 1 tablespoon
of the mixture into each cup. Refrigerate for 1 hour or more, until hard-
ened. Store in the refrigerator until ready to serve.

NOTES: Coconut butter is different from coconut oil. It's jarred, ground
coconut flesh. You can also use it as a spread, much as you would almond butter.

Fat bombs will melt if not refrigerated.

CHICKEN, BLACK BEAN, AND QUINOA POWER BOWL

PREP TIME: **20 MIN.** | COOK TIME: **10 MIN.** | YIELD: **4 SERVINGS**

CHICKEN

1 tablespoon coconut oil or avocado oil

1 pound boneless, skinless chicken breast or thighs, cut into 1-inch cubes

1 teaspoon chili powder

1/2 teaspoon garlic powder

1 teaspoon Celtic or pink Himalayan salt

1/2 teaspoon freshly ground black pepper

DRESSING

1 to 1 1/2 ripe avocados

Juice of 1 to 2 limes (3 to 4 tablespoons)

1/2 to 1 teaspoon ground cumin

1 teaspoon chili powder

Dash of cayenne pepper

THE "BOWL"

1/4 to 1/2 cup roughly chopped cilantro

About 3 cups your choice raw greens (lettuce, spinach, kale, etc.) cut into ribbons

3 cups cooked quinoa (from 1 cup dry)

1 (15-ounce) can black beans, drained and rinsed

1/4 cup pumpkin seeds, toasted

Make the chicken. Heat a large skillet over medium-high heat and add the oil.

In a medium bowl, season the chicken with the chili powder, garlic powder, salt, and black pepper. Add the seasoned chicken to the skillet and cook for 8 to 10 minutes, until chicken is fully cooked. Remove the skillet from the heat and let the chicken cool for 5 minutes.

Make the dressing. In a blender, combine all the dressing ingredients and blend until creamy. Set aside.

To build the bowl, combine the cilantro and greens and distribute evenly into four bowls. Top with the quinoa, black beans, and chicken. Drizzle the dressing evenly over each bowl and sprinkle the pumpkin seeds over the top.

BLISTERED SHISHITO PEPPERS

PREP TIME: **5 MIN.** | COOK TIME: **10 TO 15 MIN.** | YIELD: **4 SERVINGS**

1 pound shishito peppers

2 tablespoons coconut oil or avocado oil

Flaky or coarse salt

1/2 teaspoon togarashi (see Notes; optional)

Wash and carefully dry the peppers.

In a large wide skillet, heat the oil over medium heat until hot but not smoking. Add the peppers, tossing frequently, until they begin to char and blister, 10 to 15 minutes. The peppers should not become completely charred.

Place the peppers on paper towels to drain, and season them with salt to taste and the togarashi, if using. Serve immediately.

NOTES: Togarashi, also called shichimi togarashi, is a Japanese mixture of spices that contains a combination of chiles, sesame seeds, nori (seaweed), orange peel, and ginger and can be found in ethnic markets, specialty spice shops, and larger grocery stores.

Shishito peppers are Japanese peppers often served with cocktails or as an appetizer. They are very mild peppers, but about one out of ten times, there will be a hot one!

SHRIMP OR CHICKEN WITH ARTICHOKE HEARTS AND OLIVES

PREP TIME: **15 MIN.** | COOK TIME: **20 MIN.** | YIELD: **4 SERVINGS**

2 tablespoons coconut oil, avocado oil, or ghee (page 147)

1/2 cup diced sweet onion

2 garlic cloves, minced

1 (28-ounce) can diced tomatoes, well drained

1 (8-ounce) can pitted and sliced black California olives

1 (15-ounce) can artichoke hearts in water, well drained and cut into quarters

1/2 cup white wine or Chicken Bone Broth (page 96)

1 1/2 pounds large shrimp, raw, peeled and deveined, or 1 1/4 pounds boneless, skinless chicken breasts, cut into 1-inch cubes

1/4 cup roughly chopped Italian parsley or fresh basil, plus more for serving (optional)

1 teaspoon Celtic or pink Himalayan salt

1/2 teaspoon freshly ground black pepper

Crushed red pepper, for serving (optional)

In a large skillet or Dutch oven, heat the oil over medium heat.

Add the onion and garlic and cook, stirring, for about 5 minutes. Add the tomatoes, olives, artichokes, and wine. Reduce the heat to low and simmer, uncovered, for 5 minutes.

Add the shrimp (or chicken) and parsley (or basil) and simmer, covered, for about 5 minutes (7 to 10 minutes for chicken). Stir in the salt and black pepper. Serve with more parsley or basil and crushed red pepper, if desired.

NOTE: Serve this dish over gluten-free pasta, zoodles (see Note, page 109), rice, or cauliflower "rice" (see Note, page 158).

SHRIMP WITH LEMON, BUTTER, GARLIC, AND BROCCOLI RABE

PREP TIME: **15 MIN.** | COOK TIME: **20 MIN.** | YIELD: **4 SERVINGS**

1¹/2 pounds large shrimp, raw, peeled and deveined

1 teaspoon Celtic or pink Himalayan salt

1 teaspoon freshly ground black pepper

¹/4 teaspoon crushed red pepper

2 tablespoons avocado oil or ghee (page 147)

1 bunch broccoli rabe, tough stems removed

2 garlic cloves, minced

Zest and juice of 1 lemon

In a medium bowl, season the shrimp with the salt, black pepper, and crushed red pepper. Set aside.

In a large skillet, heat 1 tablespoon of the oil over medium heat. Add the broccoli rabe and sauté for about 5 minutes. Transfer the broccoli rabe to a plate and add the remaining 1 tablespoon oil to the skillet.

Add the seasoned shrimp and sauté for about 2 minutes, turning the shrimp halfway through. Add the garlic and broccoli rabe and cook for another 3 to 5 minutes, uncovered, tossing once or twice. Remove from the heat, add the lemon zest and juice, and serve immediately.

NOTE: This is great served with cauliflower "rice" (see Note, page 158), rice, zoodles (see Note, page 109), or gluten-free pasta.

SPAGHETTI WITH CHICKEN, ARUGULA, AND BACON

PREP TIME: **15 MIN.** | COOK TIME: **20 MIN.** | YIELD: **4 SERVINGS**

4 ounces uncooked gluten-free spaghetti

6 strips sugar-, nitrite-, and nitrate-free bacon, diced

3/4 pound boneless, skinless chicken breast (about 2 large or 3 medium breasts), cut into 1/2-inch cubes

1/2 teaspoon Celtic or pink Himalayan salt

1/2 teaspoon freshly ground black pepper, plus more for serving

1 or 2 garlic cloves, minced

4 to 6 cups baby arugula

1/4 to 1/2 teaspoon crushed red pepper, plus more for serving

Cook the pasta according to the package instructions.

Meanwhile, in a large skillet, cook the bacon over medium-high heat, for about 8 minutes, until crispy. Remove from the pan and place on paper towels to drain. Keep the pan on the heat.

In a medium bowl, season the chicken with the salt and black pepper and add to the pan. Sauté for about 5 minutes, add the garlic, and cook, stirring, for 2 to 3 minutes more, until the chicken is fully cooked. Transfer the chicken and garlic to a plate and set aside. Reduce the heat to medium.

Pour off the excess fat from the pan, leaving about 2 tablespoons fat. Return it to the stove and add the cooked pasta, tossing well. Add the chicken, bacon, arugula, and crushed red pepper to the pasta and toss to combine. Serve with more black pepper and the crushed red pepper.

NOTES: This dish is also great with zoodles (see Note, page 109), rice, or cauliflower "rice" (see Note, page 158). If you wish to use cheese, grate any hard, aged cheese over the pasta before serving.

SPICY KALE CHIPS

PREP TIME: **10 MIN.** | COOK TIME: **15 TO 25 MIN.** | YIELD: **4 TO 6 SERVINGS**

2 bunches kale (about 10 ounces), stems removed

2 tablespoons avocado oil or coconut oil

1/4 cup raw cashews

5 tablespoons nutritional yeast

2 tablespoons tahini

1 teaspoon onion powder

1 teaspoon garlic powder

1/2 teaspoon Celtic or pink Himalayan salt

1/4 teaspoon freshly ground black pepper

Pinch of cayenne pepper

Preheat the oven to 300°F.

In a large bowl, combine the kale with the oil. Using your hands, rub the oil into the kale to soften it.

In a food processor or blender, combine the cashews, 4 tablespoons of the nutritional yeast, the tahini, and all the seasonings. Blend until a fine meal/paste forms.

Add the spice mixture to the kale and mix well until the kale is evenly coated.

Spread the kale on a rimmed baking sheet so the leaves are not touching or overlapping. You may need to bake in several batches. Sprinkle the kale with the remaining 1 tablespoon nutritional yeast.

Bake for 15 minutes, turn over each chip, and return the baking sheet to the oven. Bake for 5 to 10 minutes more, or until the chips are light brown and crispy, being careful not to let them burn. Cool and store in an airtight container. Do not refrigerate.

NOTE: Kale chips are their very best on the day they are made.

SPICY SESAME PASTA WITH ASIAN GREENS AND SHRIMP OR CHICKEN

PREP TIME: **20 MIN.** | COOK TIME: **20 MIN.** | YIELD: **4 TO 6 SERVINGS**

MARINADE

Juice of $1/2$ orange

2 teaspoons toasted sesame oil

1 tablespoon coconut aminos

1 or 2 garlic cloves, minced

1 (1-inch) knob fresh ginger, peeled and grated

3 scallions, cut into $1/2$-inch pieces

$1/4$ teaspoon crushed red pepper

$1/4$ teaspoon freshly ground white pepper

$1/2$ teaspoon Celtic or pink Himalayan salt

PASTA, PROTEIN, AND GREENS

$1^1/2$ pounds large shrimp, raw, peeled and deveined, or $1^1/4$ pounds chicken breast, cut into thin strips

4 to 6 ounces uncooked gluten-free pasta

2 tablespoons coconut oil or avocado oil

6 to 8 cups of a combination of your favorite greens (bok choy, chard, spinach, savoy or napa cabbage, broccolini, etc.)

Crushed red pepper, for serving

Toasted sesame seeds, for serving (optional)

In a medium, nonaluminum bowl or large food storage bag, combine all the marinade ingredients. Add the shrimp (or chicken) to the marinade and refrigerate for a minimum of 2 hours or up to 8 hours.

Cook the pasta according to the package directions.

In a large skillet or wok, heat the oil over medium-high heat. Add the shrimp (or chicken) along with the marinade and sauté for about 3 minutes, turning the shrimp (or chicken) to cook evenly. Add the greens and cook, uncovered, for 3 to 4 minutes, tossing once or twice. Remove from the heat and set aside.

Put the cooked pasta in a large bowl or platter. Pour the shrimp-and-greens mixture over the pasta and toss to combine. Serve with crushed red pepper and toasted sesame seeds, if desired.

NOTES: This dish is also great served with zoodles (see Note, page 109), rice, or cauliflower "rice" (see Note, page 158). It's equally good prepared with beef or pork. In addition to the greens, feel free to add any of your favorite vegetables.

SWEET POTATO HUMMUS

PREP TIME: **15 MIN. PLUS 45 MIN. TO 1 HOUR TO ROAST THE POTATOES** | YIELD:
ABOUT 3 CUPS DEPENDING ON SIZE OF SWEET POTATOES

1 or 2 large sweet potatoes (about 1 pound)

1 (15-ounce) can chickpeas, drained and rinsed

2 tablespoons sesame seed butter or tahini

1 tablespoon olive oil, avocado oil, or toasted walnut oil

$1/2$ to 1 teaspoon ground cumin

1 garlic clove, roughly chopped

$1/2$ to 1 teaspoon Celtic or pink Himalayan salt, or to taste

Pinch of cayenne pepper (optional)

Preheat the oven to 400°F.

Roast the sweet potatoes for 45 minutes to 1 hour, until very soft. Scoop the flesh out of the skins.

In a food processor, combine the chickpeas, sesame seed butter, oil, cumin, garlic, salt, and cayenne, if using. Process until fully combined and smooth.

Serve with crudités or Siete Foods grain-free tortilla chips.

NOTE: Siete Foods grain-free tortillas and tortilla chips are available at sietefoods.com.

BLACKBERRY LIME REFRESHER

PREP TIME: **5 MIN.** | YIELD: **1 SERVING**

Ice

1 1/2 ounces potato vodka

6 ounces blackberries, puréed and strained

1/4 cup fresh lime juice

1 cup berry, lime, or plain sparkling water or seltzer

Stevia (optional)

Fresh blackberries and a lime wedge, for garnish (optional)

Fill a tall glass with ice. Add the vodka. Pour in the blackberry purée and lime juice.

Fill the glass with sparkling water. Taste for sweetness, and add stevia to taste, if desired. Garnish with blackberries and a lime wedge, if desired.

FROZEN ORANGE SHAKE

PREP TIME: **5 MIN.** | YIELD: **1 SERVING**

1/2 cup (4 ounces) fresh or unsweetened store-bought orange juice

1/4 cup (2 ounces) full-fat coconut milk

1/2 packet Dr. Kellyann's Orange Cream Collagen Cooler

4 to 6 ice cubes

1 1/2 ounces potato vodka

Orange wedge, for garnish

In a blender, combine the orange juice, coconut milk, and Dr. Kellyann's Orange Cream Collagen powder. Add the ice and blend until smooth.

Pour the vodka into a short glass, add the orange mixture, stir well, and garnish with an orange wedge.

SKINNY MOSCOW MULE

PREP TIME: **5 MIN.** | YIELD: **1 SERVING**

1/2 to 1 teaspoon finely grated
    fresh ginger

Juice of 1/2 lime

11/2 ounces potato vodka

Ice

Sparkling water or seltzer

Stevia (optional)

Fresh mint and a lime wedge, for
    garnish

In a cocktail shaker, combine the ginger, lime juice, and vodka. Shake vigorously and allow the mixture to remain in the shaker for a few minutes to infuse the ginger flavor into the vodka.

Fill a copper mug or glass with ice, strain the mixture into the vessel, and top with sparkling water or seltzer. Add stevia to taste, if desired, and garnish with the mint and lime wedge.

LEAN, GREEN FIGHTIN' MACHINE

PREP TIME: **5 MIN** | YIELD: **1 SERVING**

Ice cubes made from Chicken
    Bone Broth (page 96) or
    Dr. Kellyann's Chicken Bone
    Broth or plain ice cubes

11/2 ounces potato vodka

1/2 cup Chicken Bone Broth
    (page 96) or Dr. Kellyann's
    Chicken Bone Broth

2 teaspoons fresh lime juice

6 (1/4-inch) slices cucumber

1/2 cup packed fresh spinach

2 or 3 sprigs fresh mint

1/2 small green apple

1 (1/2-inch) knob fresh ginger,
    peeled

Stevia (optional)

Mint leaves, green apple slice,
    cucumber slice, or lime
    wedge, for garnish

Fill a tall glass with the ice. Add the vodka, broth, and lime juice.

Process all the remaining ingredients through a juicer and add to the glass. Stir, taste, and add stevia to taste, if desired. Garnish with mint, a green apple slice, a cucumber slice, or a lime wedge.

TEQUILA GRAPEFRUIT FIZZ

PREP TIME: **5 MIN.** | YIELD: **1 SERVING**

Celtic or pink Himalayan salt
(optional)

Grapefruit, lemon, or lime wedge
(optional)

Ice

1¹/2 ounces tequila

1/4 cup fresh grapefruit juice

1 slice jalapeño

Lemon, lime, or grapefruit
sparkling water or seltzer

Lemon or lime wedge, for garnish
(optional)

If desired, spread a good amount of salt evenly on a small plate. Rub the grapefruit, lemon, or lime wedge around the rim of a martini glass and dip the rim in the salt to coat the edge of the glass. Set aside.

Fill a cocktail shaker half full with ice. Add the tequila, grapefruit juice, and jalapeño slice.

Cover, shake, and strain into the prepared martini glass. Top with sparkling water. Garnish with a lemon or lime wedge, if desired.

ONLINE RESOURCES

For daily support on your diet, and to help you win your battle against the "carb flu" and the "sugar demon," sign up for my encouraging daily e-mails at the Resources page on my website, drkellyann.com/gift.

On that page, you'll also find printable copies of my "Yes" foods and my Batch Cooking Plan, as well as the Ten-Day Meal Plan and Shopping Lists. In addition, there are printable versions of the "Your Daily Diet at a Glance" chart and a "Tweak Your Times" clock graphic to help you shift the timing of your eating window, if necessary.

For additional information on the benefits of shrinking your eating window, check out my "Shorter Eating Window = Slimmer, Healthier You" post on the Resources page. And for handy tips on working collagen into your diet, see "Collagen—Your Magic Elixir."

On the Resources page, I even have tips for giving yourself a beauty makeover at the same time as you're slimming your belly!

In addition, check out my online recipes at DrKellyann.com— you'll find lots more healthy, slimming meals to try when your diet is done.

Measurement Tracker

If you're interested in more than just belly fat loss, this tracker will help you measure your weight loss in other areas as well as your change in body mass index (BMI). You'll also find a printable copy of this Measurement Tracker on the Resources page of my website at drkellyann.com/gift.

START OF YOUR DIET					END OF YOUR DIET				
Weight:					Weight:				
Measurements:					Measurements:				
Biceps	Chest	Waist	Hips	Thighs	Biceps	Chest	Waist	Hips	Thighs
Current BMI:					Current BMI:				

TO CALCULATE YOUR BMI (BODY MASS INDEX):

Measure your height in inches. To do this, stand against a wall and use a pencil to make a mark at the top of your head.

Take your height in inches and square the number. (Multiply the number of inches by itself.)

Divide your weight in pounds by your height in inches squared.

Multiply the answer by 703. This is your body mass index. While this number isn't infallible, it can give you a rough idea of the amount of body fat you have. Here's a guide you can use.

BMI	Weight
Below 18.5	Underweight
18.5 to 24.9	Normal or Healthy Weight
25.0 to 29.9	Overweight
30.0 and Above	Obese

Favorite Brands

I recommend these brands for their excellent taste and quality. I add new brands frequently, so check my Resources page for new arrivals!

BONE BROTH

Dr. Kellyann's Chicken Bone Broth

Dr. Kellyann's Beef Bone Broth

Dr. Kellyann's Powdered Bone Broth

BREAD

California Country Gal, Inc., Real Bread

Julian Bakery's Paleo Wraps

Siete Foods Grain-Free Tortillas

COLLAGEN PROTEIN

Dr. Kellyann's Bone Broth Protein

Dr. Kellyann's Complete Collagen Protein

Dr. Kellyann's Orange Cream Collagen Cooler

Dr. Kellyann's Collagen Hot Cocoa

Dr. Kellyann's Collagen Coffee

Dr. Kellyann's Vanilla Collagen Creamer

Dr. Kellyann's Chocolate Coconut Collagen Fiber Bar

EQUIPMENT

AquaTru Water Filtration System

Crock-Pot

Fit & Fresh Portable Drink and Formula Mixer

Instant Pot Pressure Cooker

FERMENTED FOODS

Gold Mine Natural Food Co. Organic Raw Sauerkraut

Rejuvenative Foods Pickles, Sauerkraut, Kimchi, Vegi-Delite Zing Salad

JARRED AND CANNED FOODS

Chosen Foods Avocado Mayonnaise

Primal Kitchen Avocado Mayonnaise

Natural Value Organic Coconut Milk

Pomi Chopped Tomatoes

Amy's Kitchen Organic Mild Salsa

Native Forest Artichoke Hearts

Santa Barbara Olive Company California Large Pitted Ripe Olives

Mediterranean Organic Sundried Tomatoes in Olive Oil

Wild Planet Foods Wild Alaskan Sockeye Salmon

MEAT, EGGS, DAIRY, AND OTHER DELIVERY

ButcherBox for Meat and Poultry Delivery

Vital Choice for Seafood Delivery

Eat Wild for Meat, Eggs, and Dairy Delivery

U.S. Wellness Meats for Meat and Poultry Delivery

Thrive Market for Healthy Groceries Delivery

OILS, BUTTERS, AND ANIMAL FATS

Tropical Traditions Coconut Oil

MaraNatha Almond Butter Creamy and Almond Butter Crunchy

SunButter Sunflower Seed Spread

Nutiva Organic Extra Virgin Coconut Oil

Let's Do Organic Organic Creamed Coconut

Artisana Organic Raw Coconut Butter

Ancient Organics Eat Good Fat Ghee

Pure Indian Foods Grass-Fed Ghee

PACKAGED FOODS

Gold Mine Natural Food Co. Kelp Noodles

Crown Prince Natural Smoked Oysters in Pure Olive Oil

SAUCES

Red Boat Fish Sauce

Annie's Organic Yellow Mustard

Bragg Apple Cider Vinegar

Coconut Secret Coconut Aminos

SNACKS

Living Intentions: Gone Nuts, Rosemary, Garlic Pistachios, and Almonds

Navitas Naturals: Chocolate Powder, Cacao Nibs, and Cacao Powder

Edward & Sons Trading Co. Coconut Flakes

Bare Fuji & Reds Crunchy Apple Crisps

Brothers-All-Natural Fruit Crisps

Vermont Village Organic Unsweetened Applesauce

Alive & Radiant Kale Krunch (Quite Cheezy)

Maine Coast Sea Vegetables, Inc.: Kelp

Go Raw: Sprouted Sunflower Seeds

Siete Foods Grain-Free Chips

OTHER PREFERRED BRANDS

SeaSnax for snacks

Steve's PaleoGoods for snacks and sauces

Simply Organic for seasonings

Celtic Sea Salt for sea salt and seasonings

Applegate Farms for deli meats

Nikki's for coconut butter

Thai Kitchen coconut milk

Thrive Market for organic, natural foods and supplements

SUPPLEMENTS

Dr. Kellyann's Bellabiotic

Mighty Maca Superfoods

SHARE YOUR SUCCESS!

'm so excited that you want to lose your unhealthy, unsightly belly fat and keep it off forever. When you finish your 10-Day Belly Slimdown, let me know how it worked for you!

The official hashtag is #10daybellyslimdown. If you add this hashtag to your social media posts, my team and others looking for inspiration will be able to view your post and connect with you. You can search this hashtag on Instagram, Facebook, and Twitter and see what is being shared about the diet, including great recipe ideas.

In addition, look for me on Facebook at https://www.facebook.com/drkellyann. There you'll see a huge and *awesome* community of people who are sharing recipes, diet tips, and inspiration.

Find me on Twitter @DrKellyann and on Instagram @DrKellyannPetrucci.

ACKNOWLEDGMENTS

This book is for everyone who encouraged my revolution to help people become slimmer, younger-looking, and healthier—faster. You are so valuable in my life and so supportive of my message, and I am forever in a place of gratitude.

To my wonderful family; my beautiful friends; the *rock star* DrKellyann family; my amazing mentors; my talented colleagues; Alan Hopkins, MD, who provided invaluable medical insights; my agents; my publisher for giving me this platform; and my editor, Alyse Diamond—and to all those who believed that a rising tide lifts all boats—thank you.

There are so many behind the scenes who make me look good, and I stand in awe of your inspiring talents and constant words of encouragement.

To Dr. Mehmet Oz, for giving me the opportunity to spread my message on a national scale, and to the amazing *Dr. Oz* team—especially Jessica, for believing in me enough to say, "It's Kellyann on this one"—thank you for helping me make my dreams come true.

A special dedication to Dr. Jennifer Bonde for running DrKellyann behind the scenes for all these years. Sometimes the quiet voices are really the strongest of all.

With love and admiration.

Dr. Kellyann xoxo

NOTES

Introduction

1. H. Bays, "Adiposopathy: Is 'Sick Fat' Cardiovascular Disease?" *Journal of the American College of Cardiology* (2011), vol. 57, no. 25.

Chapter 1

1. Salk Institute for Biological Studies, "Extended Daily Fasting Overrides Harmful Effects of a High-Fat Diet: Study May Offer Drug-Free Intervention to Prevent Obesity and Diabetes," *Science Daily*, May 17, 2012; sciencedaily.com/releases/2012/05/120517131703.htm.
2. G. Reynolds, "A 12-Hour Window for a Healthy Weight," *New York Times*, January 15, 2015; well.blogs.nytimes.com/2015/01/15/a-12-hour-window-for-a-healthy-weight/?_r=1.
3. S. Gill and S. Panda, "A Smartphone App Reveals Erratic Diurnal Eating Patterns in Humans That Can Be Modulated for Health Benefits," *Cell Metabolism*, November 3, 2015, 22(5): 789–98; ncbi.nlm.nih.gov/pmc/articles/PMC4635036/.
4. University of Alabama at Birmingham, "Time-Restricted Feeding Study Shows Promise in Helping People Shed Body Fat," *Science Daily*, January 6, 2017; sciencedaily.com/releases/2017/01/170106113820.htm.
5. T. Moro et al., "Effects of Eight Weeks of Time-Restricted Feeding (16/8) on Basal Metabolism, Maximal Strength, Body Composition, Inflammation, and Cardiovascular Risk Factors in Resistance-Trained Males," *Journal*

of Translational Medicine (2016), 14: 290; ncbi.nlm.nih.gov/pmc/articles/PMC5064803/.

6. H. Chung et al., "Time-Restricted Feeding Improves Insulin Resistance and Hepatic Steatosis in a Mouse Model of Postmenopausal Obesity," *Metabolism,* December 2016, 65(12): 1743–54; ncbi.nlm.nih.gov/pubmed/27832862.

7. M. J. Duncan et al., "Restricting Feeding to the Active Phase in Middle-Aged Mice Attenuates Adverse Metabolic Effects of a High-Fat Diet," *Physiology & Behavior,* December 1, 2016, 167: 1–9; ncbi.nlm.nih.gov/pubmed/27586251.

8. "Fasting: A Trending Food Idea and a New Frontier in Longevity Science," CNBC, October 20, 2017.

9. C. Marinac et al., "Prolonged Nightly Fasting and Breast Cancer Risk: Findings from NHANES (2009–2010)," *Cancer Epidemiology, Biomarkers, and Prevention,* May 2015; cebp.aacrjournals.org/content/24/5/783.long.

10. A. W. Brown, M. M. B. Brown, and D. B. Allison, "Belief Beyond the Evidence: Using the Proposed Effect of Breakfast on Obesity to Show 2 Practices That Distort Scientific Evidence," *American Journal of Clinical Nutrition,* November 2013, vol. 98, no. 5, 1298–1308; ajcn.nutrition.org/content/98/5/1298.long.

11. Anahad O'Connor, "Myths Surround Breakfast and Weight," *New York Times,* September 10, 2013; well.blogs.nytimes.com/2013/09/10/myths-surround-breakfast-and-weight/.

12. M. Boschmann et al., "Water-Induced Thermogenesis," *Journal of Endocrinology & Metabolism* (2003), 88(12): 6015–19.

13. E. Proksch et al., "Oral Intake of Specific Bioactive Collagen Peptides Reduces Skin Wrinkles and Increases Dermal Matrix Synthesis," Skin Pharmacology and Physiology (2014), 27: 113–19; karger.com/Article/Abstract/355523.

14. M. Tanaka et al., "Effects of Collagen Peptide Ingestion on UV-B–Induced Skin Damage," *Bioscience, Biotechnology, and Biochemistry* (2009), vol. 73, iss. 4; tandfonline.com/doi/abs/10.1271/bbb.80649.

15. M. Borumand and S. Sibilla, "Daily Consumption of the Collagen Supplement Pure Gold Collagen® Reduces Visible Signs of Aging," *Clinical Interventions in Aging,* October 13, 2014; ncbi.nlm.nih.gov/pmc/articles/PMC4206255/.

16. J. Scala et al., "Effect of Daily Gelatin Ingestion on Human Scalp Hair," *Nutrition Reports,* 13, 1976; researchgate.net/publication/279548216_Effect_of_daily_gelatin_ingestion_on_human_scalp_hair.

17. J. Michaelson and D. Huntsman, "New Aspects of the Effects of Gelatin on Fingernails," *Journal of the Society of Cosmetic Chemists* (1963), vol. 14, no. 9, 443–54; journal.scconline.org/abstracts/cc1963/cc014n09/p00443-p00454.html.

18. H. Farouk et al., "Effect of Grapefruit Juice and Sibutramine on Body Weight Loss in Obese Rats," *African Journal of Pharmacy and Pharmacology,* February 2015, vol. 9(8), 265–73; academicjournals.org/journal/AJPP/article-full-text/81888CE51349.

19. J. Warner, "Blueberries May Banish Belly Fat," WebMD; webmd.com/heart/news/20090419/blueberries-may-banish-belly-fat.

20. I. Edirisinghe et al., "Strawberry Anthocyanin and Its Association with Postprandial Inflammation and Insulin," *British Journal of Nutrition,* Epub May 16, 2011; ncbi.nlm.nih.gov/pubmed/21736853.

21. C. Morimoto et al., "Anti-Obese Action of Raspberry Ketone," *Life Sciences*, May 27, 2005, 77(2), 194–204; sciencedirect.com/science/article/pii/S0024320505001281.

22. "What's New and Beneficial About Raspberries," *The World's Healthiest Foods*; whfoods.com/genpage.php?tname=foodspice&dbid=39.

23. C. D. Gardner et al., "Comparison of the Atkins, Zone, Ornish, and LEARN Diets for Change in Weight and Related Risk Factors Among Overweight Premenopausal Women: The A to Z Weight Loss Study: A Randomized Trial," *Journal of the American Medical Association*, March 2007, vol. 297, no. 9, 969–77; jamanetwork.com/journals/jama/fullarticle/205916.

24. I. Boers et al., "Favourable Effects of Consuming a Palaeolithic-Type Diet on Characteristics of the Metabolic Syndrome: A Randomized Controlled Pilot-Study," *Lipids in Health and Disease*, 2014; ncbi.nlm.nih.gov/pubmed/25304296.

25. T. Jönsson et al., "Beneficial Effects of a Paleolithic Diet on Cardiovascular Risk Factors in Type 2 Diabetes: A Randomized Cross-Over Pilot Study," *Cardiovascular Diabetology*, 2009; ncbi.nlm.nih.gov/pubmed/?term=Beneficial+effects+of+a+Paleolithic+diet+on+cardiovascular+risk+factors+in+type+2+diabetes%3A+a+randomized+cross-over+pilot+study.

26. "Low Glycaemic Index or Low Glycaemic Load Diets for Overweight and Obesity," Cochrane Collaboration (2007); cochrane.org/CD005105/ENDOC_low-glycaemic-index-or-low-glycaemic-load-diets-for-overweight-and-obesity.

27. R. Chowdhury et al., "Association of Dietary, Circulating, and Supplement Fatty Acids with Coronary Risk: A Systematic Review and Meta-Analysis," *Annals of Internal Medicine*, March 18, 2014, 160(6): 398–406; ncbi.nlm.nih.gov/pubmed/24723079.

28. Russell J. deSouza et al., "Intake of Saturated and Trans Unsaturated Fatty Acids and Risk of All Cause Mortality, Cardiovascular Disease, and Type 2 Diabetes: Systematic Review and Meta-Analysis of Observational Studies," *British Medical Journal*, August 2015 (online); bmj.com/content/351/bmj.h3978/.

29. M. L. Assunção et al., "Effects of Dietary Coconut Oil on the Biochemical and Anthropometric Profiles of Women Presenting Abdominal Obesity," *Lipids*, July 2009, 44(7): 593–601; ncbi.nlm.nih.gov/pubmed/19437058.

30. H. Müller et al., "A Diet Rich in Coconut Oil Reduces Diurnal Postprandial Variations in Circulating Tissue Plasminogen Activator Antigen and Fasting Lipoprotein (a) Compared with a Diet Rich in Unsaturated Fat in Women," *Journal of Nutrition*, November 2003, 133(11): 3422–27; ncbi.nlm.nih.gov/pubmed/14608053.

31. D. A. Cardoso et al., "A Coconut Extra Virgin Oil–Rich Diet Increases HDL Cholesterol and Decreases Waist Circumference and Body Mass in Coronary Artery Disease Patients," *Nutricion Hospitalaria*, November 1, 2015, 32(5): 2144–52; ncbi.nlm.nih.gov/pubmed/26545671.

32. "Does Saturated Fat Clog Your Arteries? Controversial Paper Says 'No,'" CNN, April 27, 2017; cnn.com/2017/04/25/health/saturated-fat-arteries-study/index.html.

33. M. Daimon et al., "Decreased Serum Levels of Adiponectin Are a Risk Factor for the Progression to Type 2 Diabetes in the Japanese Population," *Diabetes Care* (2003), 26: 2015–20.

34. M. Kumada et al., "Association of Hypoadiponectinemia with Coronary Artery Disease in Men," *Arteriosclerosis, Thrombosis, and Vascular Biology* (2003), 23: 35–39.

Chapter 2

1. "Black Pepper Fights Formation of Fat Cells," UPI, May 7, 2012; upi.com/Health_News/2012/05/07/Black-pepper-fights-formation-of-fat-cells/UPI-20801336435628/#ixzz1uHsvZGNI.
2. L. M. Nackers et al., "The Association Between Rate of Initial Weight Loss and Long-Term Success in Obesity Treatment: Does Slow and Steady Win the Race?" *International Journal of Behavioral Medicine*, September 2010, 17(3): 161–67; link.springer.com/article/10.1007%2Fs12529-010-9092-y.
3. A. Carroll, "Behind New Dietary Guidelines, Better Science," *New York Times*, February 23, 2015.
4. A. Abbott, "Sugar Substitutes Linked to Obesity," *Nature News*, September 17, 2014; nature.com/news/sugar-substitutes-linked-to-obesity-1.15938.
5. J. A. Monro, R. Leon, and B. K. Puri, "The Risk of Lead Contamination in Bone Broth Diets," *Medical Hypotheses*, April 2013, 80(4): 389–90.
6. Original report accessed from drkaayladaniel.com/boning-up-is-broth-contaminated-with-lead/.
7. M. J. Baxter et al., "Lead Contamination During Domestic Preparation and Cooking of Potatoes and Leaching of Bone-Derived Lead on Roasting, Marinading, and Boiling Beef," *Food Additives and Contaminants*, May–June 1992, 9(3): 225–35.

Chapter 3

1. Y. Wang et al., "Will All Americans Become Overweight or Obese? Estimating the Progression and Cost of the US Obesity Epidemic," *Obesity*, October 2008, 16(10): 2323–30; onlinelibrary.wiley.com/doi/10.1038/oby.2008.351/full.
2. R. Noordam et al., "High Serum Glucose Levels Are Associated with a Higher Perceived Age," *Age*, February 2013, 35(1): 189–95.
3. D. B. Samadi, "Study Links Sugar to Cancer: How to Reduce Your Risk," Fox News, January 6, 2016.
4. "Is Sugar Making Us Sick?" *Berkeley Wellness*, August 3, 2015.
5. J. Norris, "Sugared Soda Consumption, Cell Aging Associated in New Study," UCSF News, October 16, 2014.

Chapter 6

1. S. Reardon, "Food Preservatives Linked to Obesity and Gut Disease," *Nature News*, February 25, 2015; nature.com/news/food-preservatives-linked-to-obesity-and-gut-disease-1.16984.

2. H. Parker, "A Sweet Problem: Princeton Researchers Find That High-Fructose Corn Syrup Prompts Considerably More Weight Gain," Princeton University News, March 22, 2010; princeton.edu/main/news/archive/S26/91/22K07/.

3. K. Lau et al., "Synergistic Interactions Between Commonly Used Food Additives in a Developmental Neurotoxicity Test," *Toxicological Sciences* (2006), 90(1): 178–87.

Chapter 7

1. M-P St-Onge and P. J. H. Jones, "Physiological Effects of Medium-Chain Triglycerides: Potential Agents in the Prevention of Obesity," *Journal of Nutrition,* March 1, 2002, 132(3): 329–32; jn.nutrition.org/content/132/3/329.full.

2. Berta Buey et al. "Comparative Effect of Bovine Buttermilk, Whey, and Lactoferrin on the Innate Immunity Receptors and Oxidative Status of Intestinal Epithelial Cells," *Biochemistry and Cell Biology,* June 13, 2020 (online), https://pubmed.ncbi.nlm.nih.gov/32538128/.

3. Ágnes A. Fekete et al. "Whey Protein Lowers Blood Pressure And Improves Endothelial Function and Lipid Biomarkers in Adults with Prehypertension and Mild Hypertension: Results from the Chronic Whey2Go Randomized Controlled Trial," *American Journal of Clinical Nutrition,* 104(6), December 2016, 1534–44, https://pubmed.ncbi.nlm.nih.gov/27797709/.

4. Sebely Pal et al. "Effects of Whey Protein Isolate on Body Composition, Lipids, Insulin and Glucose in Overweight and Obese Individuals," *British Journal of Nutrition,* 104(5), September 2010, 716–23, https://pubmed.ncbi.nlm.nih.gov/20377924/.

Chapter 8

1. M. A. M. Rogers and D. M. Aronoff, "The Influence of Non-Steroidal Anti-Inflammatory Drugs on the Gut Microbiome," *Clinical Microbiology and Infection,* February 2016, 22(2): 178.e1–178.e9; clinicalmicrobiologyandinfection.com/article/S1198-743X(15)00902-7/fulltext?cc=y=.

Chapter 9

1. M. Bhasin et al., "Relaxation Response Induces Temporal Transcriptome Changes in Energy Metabolism, Insulin Secretion and Inflammatory Pathways," *PLOS ONE,* May 1, 2013; journals.plos.org/plosone/article?id=10.1371/journal.pone.0062817.

2. R. Rettner, "The Truth About '10,000 Steps a Day,'" *Live Science;* livescience.com/43956-walking-10000-steps-healthy.html.

3. F. Maillard et al., "High-Intensity Interval Training Reduces Abdominal Fat Mass in Postmenopausal Women with Type 2 Diabetes," *Diabetes & Metabolism,* August 24, 2016, 42(6): 433–41; diabet-metabolism.com/article/S1262-3636(16)30470-0/fulltext?cc=y=.

4. M. Heydari, J. Freund, and S. H. Boutcher, "The Effect of High-Intensity Intermittent Exercise on Body Composition of Overweight Young Males," *Journal of Obesity*, 2012 (online); hindawi.com/journals/jobe/2012/480467/.

5. "Embrace the Cold: Evidence That Shivering and Exercise May Convert White Fat to Brown," *Science Daily*, February 4, 2014; sciencedaily.com/releases/2014/02/140204123619.htm.

6. Nicky Phillips, "Forget the Jog Slog and Fit in a Sprint for Maximum Weight Loss Results," *Executive Style*, June 29, 2012; executivestyle.com.au/forget-the-jog-slog-and-fit-in-a-sprint-for-maximum-weight-loss-results-215a4.

7. M. Lowery, "Why Exercising on an Empty Stomach Is the Secret to Weight Loss," *The Telegraph*, June 13, 2017; telegraph.co.uk/health-fitness/body/exercising-empty-stomach-secret-weight-loss/?WT.mc_id=tmg_share_em.

8. I. Diaz et al., "Effects of Resistance Training on Obese Adolescents," *Medicine and Science in Sports and Exercise*, December 2015, 47(12): 2636–44; ncbi.nlm.nih.gov/pubmed/25973557.

9. B. S. Shaw et al., "Anthropometric and Cardiovascular Responses to Hypertrophic Resistance Training in Postmenopausal Women," *Menopause*, November 2016, 23(11): 1176–81; ncbi.nlm.nih.gov/pubmed/27433861.

10. S. Tsuzuku et al., "Favorable Effects of Non-Instrumental Resistance Training on Fat Distribution and Metabolic Profiles in Healthy Elderly People," *European Journal of Applied Physiology*, March 2007, 99(5): 549–55; link.springer.com/article/10.1007/s00421-006-0377-4.

11. M. Lally, "Why Your Handbag Is Making You Fat (and So Are Your Fake Tan, High Heels and Leggings!)," *Daily Mail*, April 22, 2012; dailymail.co.uk/femail/article-2133575/Why-handbag-making-fat-And-fake-tan-high-heels-leggings.html.

12. R. Beever, "Do 'Far-Infrared' Saunas Have Cardiovascular Benefits in People with Type II Diabetes Mellitis? A Sequential Longitudinal Interrupted Time Series Design Study"; sunlighten.com/wp-content/uploads/2016/09/Dr-Beever-Weight-Loss-Research.pdf.

Chapter 10

1. "Mindfulness Meditation Is Associated with Structural Changes in the Brain," National Center for Complementary and Integrative Health; nccih.nih.gov/research/results/spotlight/012311.htm.

2. "Yoga for Anxiety and Depression," *Chicago Tribune*, September 16, 2009.

3. C. Wang et al., "Tai Chi on Psychological Well-Being: Systematic Review and Meta-Analysis," *BMC Complementary and Alternative Medicine*, May 21, 2010 (online); bmccomplementalternmed.biomedcentral.com/articles/10.1186/1472-6882-10-23.

4. J. Easton, "Sleep Loss Boosts Hunger and Unhealthy Food Choice," *UChicago News*, March 1, 2016.

5. K. L. Knutson, "Impact of Sleep and Sleep Loss on Glucose Homeostasis and Appetite Regulation," *Sleep Medicine Clinics*, June 2007, 2(2): 187–97; ncbi.nlm.nih.gov/pmc/articles/PMC2084401/.

6. C. Olley, "The Wrong Light Could Be Making You Fat," *Rodale Wellness*, June 9, 2014; rodalewellness.com/health/blue-light-and-weight-gain.

Chapter 11

1. "Body Burden: Findings and Recommendations," Environmental Working Group; ewg.org/sites/bodyburden1/findings.php.

2. F. MacDonald, "BPA Exposure Has Been Linked to an Increase in Diabetes and Obesity," *Science Alert*, September 29, 2015; sciencealert.com/bpa-exposure-has-been-linked-to-increases-in-diabetes-and-obesity.

3. Cited in O. A. H. Jones et al., "Environmental Pollution and Diabetes: A Neglected Association," *The Lancet*, January 26, 2008; thelancet.com/article/S0140-6736(08)60147-6/abstract.

4. S. Begley, "Study: Air Pollution Heightens Risk of Obesity and Diabetes," *Time*, February 22, 2016; time.com/4233241/air-pollution-obesity-diabetes/.

5. Jean-Philippe Bastard and Bruno Feve, *Physiology and Physiopathology of Adipose Tissue* (New York: Springer, 2012).

6. O. Hue, O. J. Marcotte, F. Berrigan, et al., "Increased Plasma Levels of Toxic Pollutants Accompanying Weight Loss Induced by Hypocaloric Diet or by Bariatric Surgery," *Obesity Surgery* (2006), 16: 1145–54; link.springer.com/article/10.1381%2F096089206778392356.

7. C. Casals-Casas et al., "Endocrine Disruptors: From Endocrine to Metabolic Disruption," *Annual Review of Physiology* (2011), 73: 135–62; annualreviews.org/doi/abs/10.1146/annurev-physiol-012110-142200?url_ver=Z39.88-2003&rfr_dat=cr_pub%3Dpubmed&rfr_id=ori%3Arid%3Acrossref.org&journalCode=physiol.

8. "Energy Balance and Pollution by Organochlorines and Polychlorinated Biphenyls," ncbi.nlm.nih.gov/pubmed/12608524.

9. "Toxicological Function of Adipose Tissue: Focus on Persistent Organic Pollutants"; ncbi.nlm.nih.gov/pmc/articles/PMC3569688/pdf/ehp.1205485.pdf.

10. "Adipocytes Under Assault: Environmental Disruption of Adipose Physiology"; ncbi.nlm.nih.gov/pmc/articles/PMC3823640/pdf/nihms495984.pdf.

11. "Environmental Obesogens: Organotins and Endocrine Disruption via Nuclear Receptor Signaling;" academic.oup.com/endo/article-lookup/doi/10.1210/en.2005-1129.

12. "Toxicological Function of Adipose Tissue: Focus on Persistent Organic Pollutants"; ncbi.nlm.nih.gov/pmc/articles/PMC3569688/pdf/ehp.1205485.pdf.

13. "EPA Addressing the Use of Persistent Organic Pollutants"; epa.gov/international-cooperation/persistent-organic-pollutants-global-issue-global-response#thedirtydozen.

14. Stockholm Convention; pops.int/.

15. C. Casals-Casas et al., "Endocrine Disruptors: From Endocrine to Metabolic Disruption"; annualreviews.org/doi/abs/10.1146/annurev-physiol-012110-142200?url_ver=Z39.88-2003&rfr_dat=cr_pub%3Dpubmed&rfr_id=ori%3Arid%3Acrossref.org&journalCode=physiol.

16. World Health Organization PowerPoint on POPs: who.int/ceh/capacity/POPs.pdf.

17. M. Blake, "The Scary New Evidence on BPA-Free Plastics," *Mother Jones*, March/April 2014; motherjones.com/environment/2014/03/tritan-certichem-eastman-bpa-free-plastic-safe/.

18. K. Feldscher, "Unsafe Levels of Toxic Chemicals Found in Drinking Water of 33 States," *Harvard Gazette*, August 9, 2016; news.harvard.edu/gazette/story/2016/08/unsafe-levels-of-toxic-chemicals-found-in-drinking-water-of-33-states/.

19. National Tap Water Quality Database, Environmental Working Group; ewg.org/agmag/2005/12/national-tap-water-quality-database.

20. O. Milman and J. Glenza, "At Least 33 U.S. Cities Used Water Testing 'Cheats' over Lead Concerns," *The Guardian*, June 2, 2016; theguardian.com/environment/2016/jun/02/lead-water-testing-cheats-chicago-boston-philadelphia.

21. State of American Drinking Water, Environmental Working Group; ewg.org/tapwater/state-of-american-drinking-water.php.

Chapter 13

1. M. D. Klok et al., "The Role of Leptin and Ghrelin in the Regulation of Food Intake and Body Weight in Humans: A Review," *Obesity Reviews*, January 2007, 8(1): 21–34; ncbi.nlm.nih.gov/pubmed/17212793.

2. "Researchers Identify Cause of Insulin Resistance in Type 2 Diabetics," *Science Daily*, March 7, 2016; sciencedaily.com/releases/2016/03/160307113548.htm.

3. M. I. Schmidt et al., "Markers of Inflammation and Prediction of Diabetes Mellitus in Adults (Atherosclerosis Risk in Communities Study): A Cohort Study," *The Lancet*, May 15, 1999, 353(9165): 1649–52; thelancet.com/journals/lancet/article/PIIS0140-6736(99)01046-6/abstract.

4. "Prediabetes & Insulin Resistance," National Institute of Diabetes and Digestive and Kidney Diseases; niddk.nih.gov/health-information/diabetes/types/prediabetes-insulin-resistance.

5. M. Cappel et al., "Correlation Between Serum Levels of Insulin-like Growth Factor 1, Dehydroepiandrosterone Sulfate, and Dihydrotestosterone and Acne Lesion Counts in Adult Women," *JAMA Dermatology* (2005), 141(3): 333–38; archderm.jamanetwork.com/article.aspx?articleid=393279&resultclick=1.

6. S. E. Shoelson et al., "Inflammation and Insulin Resistance," *Journal of Clinical Investigation*, July 3, 2006, 116(7): 1793–1801; ncbi.nlm.nih.gov/pmc/articles/PMC1483173/.

7. L. H. Wyatt et al., "The Musculoskeletal Effects of Diabetes Mellitus," *Journal of the Canadian Chiropractic Association*, March 2006, 50(1); ncbi.nlm.nih.gov/pmc/articles/PMC1839979/.

8. A. Laws and G. M. Reaven, "Evidence for an Independent Relationship Between Insulin Resistance and Fasting Plasma HDL-Cholesterol, Triglyceride and Insulin Concentrations," *Journal of Internal Medicine*, January 1992; onlinelibrary.wiley.com/doi/10.1111/j.1365-2796.1992.tb00494.x/full.

9. A. Salvetti et al., "The Inter-Relationship Between Insulin Resistance and Hypertension," *Drugs*, 1993, Suppl. 2: 149–59; ncbi.nlm.nih.gov/pubmed/7512468.

10. J. Maljaars et al., "Effect of Fat Saturation on Satiety, Hormone Release, and Food Intake," *American Journal of Clinical Nutrition*, April 2009, 89(4): 1019–24; ajcn.nutrition.org/content/89/4/1019.full.

11. K. Nagao and T. Yanagita, "Medium-Chain Fatty Acids: Functional Lipids for the Prevention and Treatment of the Metabolic Syndrome," *Pharmacological Research*, March 2010, 61(3): 208–12; ncbi.nlm.nih.gov/pubmed/19931617.

12. H. Kaunitz, "Medium Chain Triglycerides (MCT) in Aging and Arterio-sclerosis," *Europe PMC* (1986), 6(3–4): 115–21; europepmc.org/abstract/med/3519928.

13. R. J. Stubbs et al., "The Effect of Covertly Manipulating the Energy Density of Mixed Diets on Ad Libitum Food Intake in 'Pseudo Free-Living' Humans," *International Journal of Obesity and Related Metabolic Disorders*, October 1998, 22(10): 980–87; ncbi.nlm.nih.gov/pubmed/9806313.

14. J. Maljaars et al., "Effect of Fat Saturation on Satiety, Hormone Release, and Food Intake," *American Journal of Clinical Nutrition*, April 2009, 89(4): 1019–24; ajcn.nutrition.org/content/89/4/1019.full.

15. A. Himaya et al., "Satiety Power of Dietary Fat: A New Appraisal," *American Journal of Clinical Nutrition*, May 1997, vol. 65, no. 5, 1410–18; ajcn.nutrition.org/content/65/5/1410.abstract.

16. X. Y. Qi et al., "Mogrosides Extract from Siraitia Grosvenori Scavenges Free Radicals in Vitro and Lowers Oxidative Stress, Serum Glucose, and Lipid Levels in Alloxan-Induced Diabetic Mice," *Nutrition Research*, April 2008, 28(4): 278–84; sciencedirect.com/science/article/pii/S0271531708000365.

INDEX

Also available from

KELLYANN PETRUCCI,
MS, ND

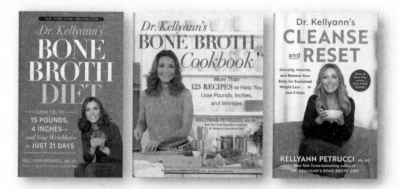

"Dr. Kellyann is a leader in the weight-loss and anti-aging fields, and she knows her stuff."

—ANTHONY YOUN, MD, FACS, America's Holistic Plastic Surgeon™ and author of *The Age Fix*

RODALE
BOOKS

Available wherever books are sold